Department of Veterans Affairs
Health Services Research & Development Service

Evidence-based Synthesis Program

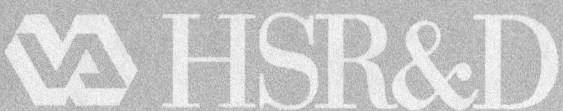

Performance Characteristics of Self-report Instruments for Diagnosing Generalized Anxiety and Panic Disorders in Primary Care: A Systematic Review

I0470816

August 2011

Prepared for:
Department of Veterans Affairs
Veterans Health Administration
Health Services Research & Development Service
Washington, DC 20420

Prepared by:
Evidence-based Synthesis Program (ESP) Center
Durham Veterans Affairs Healthcare System
Durham, N.C.
John W. Williams Jr., M.D., M.H.Sc, Director

Investigators:
Principal Investigator:
Sophiya Benjamin, M.D.

Co-Investigators:
Nathaniel R. Herr, Ph.D.
Jennifer McDuffie, Ph.D.
John W. Williams Jr., M.D., M.H.Sc

Research Associate:
Avishek Nagi, M.S.

Medical Editor:
Liz Wing, M.A.

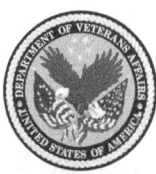

PREFACE

Health Services Research & Development Service's (HSR&D's) Evidence-based Synthesis Program (ESP) was established to provide timely and accurate syntheses of targeted healthcare topics of particular importance to Veterans Affairs (VA) managers and policymakers, as they work to improve the health and healthcare of Veterans. The ESP disseminates these reports throughout VA.

HSR&D provides funding for four ESP Centers and each Center has an active VA affiliation. The ESP Centers generate evidence syntheses on important clinical practice topics, and these reports help:

- develop clinical policies informed by evidence,
- guide the implementation of effective services to improve patient outcomes and to support VA clinical practice guidelines and performance measures, and
- set the direction for future research to address gaps in clinical knowledge.

In 2009, the ESP Coordinating Center was created to expand the capacity of HSR&D Central Office and the four ESP sites by developing and maintaining program processes. In addition, the Center established a Steering Committee comprised of HSR&D field-based investigators, VA Patient Care Services, Office of Quality and Performance, and Veterans Integrated Service Networks (VISN) Clinical Management Officers. The Steering Committee provides program oversight, guides strategic planning, coordinates dissemination activities, and develops collaborations with VA leadership to identify new ESP topics of importance to Veterans and the VA healthcare system.

Comments on this evidence report are welcome and can be sent to Nicole Floyd, ESP Coordinating Center Program Manager, at nicole.floyd@va.gov.

Recommended citation: Benjamin S, Herr NR, McDuffie J, Nagi A, Williams JW Jr. Performance Characteristics of Self-report Instruments for Diagnosing Generalized Anxiety and Panic Disorders in Primary Care: A Systematic Review. VA-ESP Project #09-010; 2011

TABLE OF CONTENTS

EXECUTIVE SUMMARY

BACKGROUND

Generalized anxiety disorder (GAD) and panic disorder (PD) are two common mental illnesses that present in primary care clinics, often with physical symptoms that can inhibit appropriate diagnosis and treatment. Recognition of these disorders by primary care physicians is much lower than the expected rates—in part due to somatic presentations but also due to the lack of routine screening that is in place for some other mental illnesses. Patients with anxiety disorders are often high utilizers of health care resources, and when their anxiety disorders are not diagnosed and treated, they can frequently undergo more expensive testing to rule out medical causes.

Identification of accurate and feasible screening instruments for GAD and PD that have been validated in primary care settings have the potential to improve detection and facilitate treatment of these disorders within the primary care clinic, or to generate appropriate referral. Our report is a systematic review of the literture to evaluate the performance of self-report instruments used to diagnose GAD and PD in primary care settings.

Three key questions (KQs) guided this systematic review:

KQ 1. In general medical patients with somatic symptoms, what are the performance characteristics (e.g., sensitivity, specificity) of self-report questionnaires for diagnosing generalized anxiety disorder or panic disorder?

KQ 2. For questionnaires evaluated in KQ 1, which measures are most feasible to use in primary care settings? Specifically, what is the reading comprehension level, time required to complete, response format, and compatibility with telephone administration?

KQ 3. For questionnaires evaluated in KQ 1, do the performance characteristics vary by gender, race, age group, or setting?

METHODS

We searched PubMed® from 1980 to 2010 using standard search terms. We searched for primary studies and systematic reviews in MEDLINE® (via PubMed), PsycINFO®, and the Cochrane Library. We limited the search to peer-reviewed articles involving adult human subjects and published in the English language. Additional citations were identified from reference lists of articles included at the full-text review level. Titles, abstracts, and articles were reviewed in duplicate by investigators trained in the critical analysis of literature. Data were extracted by quantitative analysts. Pooled analyses were performed when appropriate. All other data were narratively summarized.

Study characteristics, patient characteristics, and outcomes were extracted by trained research staff under the supervision of the Program Director. We assessed study quality according to the Quality Assessment of Diagnostic Accuracy Studies (QUADAS) criteria modified for this specific research question.

DATA SYNTHESIS

We constructed evidence tables showing study, patient, and intervention characteristics; methodological quality; and outcomes, organized by key question. We analyzed studies to compare their characteristics, methods, and findings. We compiled a summary of findings for each question based on qualitative and semiquantitative synthesis of the findings and provided a final assessment of the current evidence based on the Grades of Recommendation, Assessment, Development, and Evaluation (GRADE) Working Group criteria.

PEER REVIEW

A draft version of the report was reviewed by technical experts as well as clinical leadership, and their comments are provided in the appendix.

RESULTS

We screened 2890 titles, rejected 2824, and performed a more detailed review of 66 articles. From these, we identified no recent systematic reviews and 12 observational reports on 9 unique studies that addressed one of the key questions.

KQ 1. In general medical patients with somatic symptoms, what are the performance characteristics (e.g., sensitivity, specificity) of self-report questionnaires for diagnosing generalized anxiety disorder or panic disorder?

We identified eight screening instruments for the detection of GAD and PD in primary care patients. Of these, the Generalized Anxiety Disorder-7 (GAD-7; sensitivity 89%, specificity 82%) and the panic module of the Patient Health Questionnaire (PHQ; sensitivity 80%, specificity 99%) had the best performance characteristics for the diagnosis of GAD and PD, respectively. The Symptom Driven Diagnostic System–Primary Care (SDDS-PC) also had good performance characteristics and is a multicomponent instrument that screens for GAD and PD as well as other mental illnesses.

All of the above instruments have been evaluated in reasonably sized primary care populations; however, none of these studies have been rigorously replicated. Even the SDDS-PC instrument that was evaluated in two studies consisted of two different versions. Therefore, evidence for these instruments is based on a single, well-conducted study for each instrument. Heterogeneity among the studies was high, prohibiting statistical pooling of data except in the case of some performance characteristics for the SDDS-PC.

Though KQ 1 addressed anxiety screening instruments in primary care populations with somatic symptoms, the samples in the studies identified were unselected and were seeing their primary care physician for a variety of complaints including routine followup. The instruments may perform differently in this setting when compared to a case-finding model where the same instrument is applied to patients with specific somatic complaints associated with a higher risk of having GAD or PD. We identified only one study that screened such patients, who were evaluated for palpitations.

KQ 2. For questionnaires evaluated in KQ 1, which measures are most feasible to use in primary care settings? Specifically, what is the reading comprehension level, time required to complete, response format, and compatibility with telephone administration?

There was limited evidence addressing the feasibility of using these instruments in primary care. The evidence was qualitative and indirectly inferred from the primary studies.

The instruments were 3 to 11 questions in length and were at an easy to average reading level. Across the four studies reporting administration times, most patients completed the instrument in less than 2 minutes.

There was no evidence to assess the validity of these instruments for telephone administration though some trials have already used instruments like the Primary Care Evaluation of Mental Disorders (PRIME-MD) via telephone. None of the instruments have been studied specifically for responsiveness to change in symptoms status.

KQ 3. For questionnaires evaluated in KQ 1, do the performance characteristics vary by gender, race, age group, or setting?

Only one of the studies formally assessed differences in performance characteristics by race. When the Brief Panic Disorder Scale (BPDS) was administered to a biracial population, it performed better among Caucasians at the traditional cutoff of 10. The instrument was more specific among Caucasians and resulted in more false positives among African Americans. Thus, there is preliminary evidence that instruments might perform differently among different racial and ethnic groups.

None of the studies addressed differences in performance based on gender, age, or setting.

FUTURE RESEARCH

Based on study quality, operating characteristics, precision of the estimates, potential for assessing response to change, and other feasibility issues, the most promising instruments are: the panic module of the PHQ, the GAD-7 and the SDDS-PC. Future studies should focus on replicating the results of performance characteristics of these instruments, specifically in Veterans Affairs (VA) samples as we did not find any rigorous validation of any instruments in this review in the Veterans Health Administration (VHA) system. These studies should also incorporate questions of feasibility, such as time taken to complete, acceptability among patients, and sensitivity to change. Finally, results should be analyzed by race, gender, setting, and age to explore possible differences in performance of the instruments based on these variables.

ABBREVIATIONS TABLE

BPDS	Brief Panic Disorder Scale
GAD	generalized anxiety disorder
GRADE	Grades of Recommendation, Assessment, Development, and Evaluation
KQ	key question
PD	panic disorder
PHQ	Patient Health Questionnaire
PRIME-MD	Primary Care Evaluation of Mental Disorders
QUADAS	Quality Assessment of Diagnostic Accuracy Studies
SDDS-PC	Symptom Driven Diagnostic System–Primary Care
VA	Veterans Affairs
VHA	Veterans Health Administration

EVIDENCE REPORT

INTRODUCTION

Anxiety disorders are a major public health concern associated with functional impairment and increased use of the health care system.[1,2] Two of the more common anxiety disorders are generalized anxiety disorder (GAD) and panic disorder (PD), which if identified, can be treated successfully with medications or psychotherapy. GAD is characterized by at least 6 months of persistent and excessive anxiety and worry that is difficult to control and is accompanied by three of six additional symptoms: restlessness, fatigue, decreased concentration, irritability, muscle tension, and sleep disturbance.[3] PD, on the other hand, is episodic in nature and characterized by recurrent and unexpected panic attacks—periods of intense fear or terror associated with autonomic arousal such as breathlessness, chest pain, or fear of losing control—that become a cause of persistent concern in the patient.[3]

In community samples, GAD has a lifetime prevalence of 5.1 percent in the U.S. population aged 15 to 54 years.[4] The prevalence of PD in the National Comorbidity Survey was 2.3 percent in the 12-month period prior to the interview and 3.5 percent over one's lifetime.[5] The same study found that in the 12-month period preceding the interview, anxiety disorders (17%) were more likely to occur when compared to other common mental illnesses such as substance abuse (11%) and affective disorders (11%), indicating that anxiety disorders are more chronic in nature.[5] In the sample of participants aged 55 years or older, the 12-month prevalence of GAD was 2 percent, and PD was found to be 1.3 percent.[6] The prevalence of these disorders in primary care populations is higher than in community samples, with rates for GAD at 7.6 percent and PD at 6.8 percent.[7]

Among Operation Enduring Freedom and Operation Iraqi Freedom (OEF/OIF) Veterans referred for further behavioral health assessment based on preliminary screening, the incidence for GAD was 4.2 percent and for PD, 8 percent. Further, both disorders were significantly associated with limitations on work performance across multiple domains, thus affecting a Veteran's ability to maintain gainful employment and successfully reintegrate into civilian life.[8] The main barrier to receiving mental health treatment among Veterans is stigma: 65 percent of Veterans who met screening criteria for a mental disorder stated, "I would be seen as weak."[9] Besides stigma-related reasons, more pragmatic concerns, such as difficulty scheduling appointments or getting time off from work, were high on the list.[9]

BACKGROUND

Many patients with anxiety disorders present to their primary care doctors.[7] However, almost half of the patients with an anxiety disorder are not diagnosed or treated. One obstacle in the diagnosis of anxiety disorders is the somatic presentation.[10,11] In addition to anxiety and worry, the DSM-IV TR (text revision) includes symptoms such as restlessness, being easily fatigued, muscle tension, and sleep disturbance as diagnostic criteria for GAD—symptoms that might be associated with other common physical illnesses.[3] Similarly, the DSM-IV TR defines a panic attack as a discrete period of discomfort where 4 out of 13 symptoms are present; however, many of these symptoms—palpitations, sweating, trembling or shaking, shortness of breath, feeling of choking, chest pain or discomfort, nausea or abdominal distress, feeling dizzy, unsteady, lightheaded or faint, paresthesias, chills or hot flushes—could be considered symptoms of other medical illnesses. In the Veteran population, symptoms of GAD and PD might also be present in patients with other mental illnesses such as substance abuse, PTSD, and depression. As one author describes, anxiety is a relatively easy symptom to elicit in medical settings; the diagnostic difficulty lies in the interpretation.[12] In addition to identifying anxiety disorders that may present with physical symptoms, screening and treatment have the potential to improve patient outcomes.

Many of the barriers to the recognition, diagnosis, and effective treatment of GAD and PD parallel the quality gaps identified in the management of patients with depressive disorders.[13,14] Over the past decade, models of care that included screening and integration between primary care and mental health professionals have been shown to improve outcomes for patients with depression or anxiety disorders.[15-17] The VA has embraced these integrated-care models and employs systematic screening for depression, posttraumatic stress disorder, and alcohol-related disorders. Patients referred to the integrated-care programs are also screened for comorbid conditions, including anxiety disorders. Patients with comorbid conditions (e.g., major depressive disorder and GAD) have a more chronic course of illness and may require more intensive treatment to achieve remission.

While there exist standard screening instruments for depression (e.g., the Patient Health Questionnaire [PHQ-9][18]) and alcohol consumption (e.g., AUDIT-C[19]), there is no one instrument recommended to screen for common anxiety disorders. A uniform approach to screening for anxiety could facilitate, at a national level, the performance measurement, cross-facility comparison, and quality improvement efforts of the VA health system. Selection of a single instrument should consider evidence on performance characteristics, ease of use, and ability to monitor treatment response.[16,20-22] Instruments easiest to use in busy primary care settings will be in a self-report format and will not require specialized equipment or trained personnel, making them more feasible to implement. To inform decisionmaking regarding a standard screening instrument for anxiety disorders, we conducted a systematic review of the literature to evaluate the performance of self-report instruments used to diagnose GAD and PD in primary care settings.

METHODS

TOPIC DEVELOPMENT

This review was commissioned by the VA's Evidence-based Synthesis Program. The topic was nominated after a formal topic nomination and prioritization process that included representatives from the VA Office of Mental Health Services, Health Services Research and Development, Mental Health QUERI, and Primary Care–Mental Health Integration Program. We further developed and refined the key questions (KQs) for this review based on a preliminary review of published peer-reviewed literature in consultation with VA and non-VA experts to select patients, measures, outcomes, and settings addressed in this review.

The final KQs were:

KQ 1. In general medical patients with somatic symptoms, what are the performance characteristics (e.g., sensitivity, specificity) of self-report questionnaires for diagnosing generalized anxiety disorder or panic disorder?

KQ 2. For questionnaires evaluated in KQ 1, which measures are most feasible to use in primary care settings? Specifically, what is the reading comprehension level, time required to complete, response format, and compatibility with telephone administration?

KQ 3. For questionnaires evaluated in KQ 1, do the performance characteristics vary by gender, race, age group, or setting?

ANALYTIC FRAMEWORK

We developed and followed a standard protocol for all steps of this review. Our approach was guided by the analytic framework shown in Figure 1.

Figure 1. Analytic framework

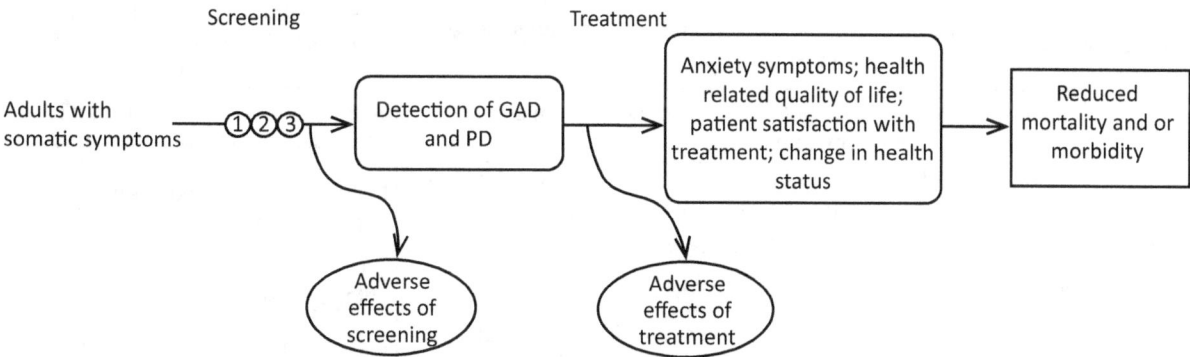

SEARCH STRATEGY

We searched MEDLINE® (via PubMed®), PsycINFO®, and the Cochrane Library for studies comparing self-report measures of GAD and PD with an acceptable criterion standard from January 1980 through December 2010. We chose 1980 to coincide with the publication of DSM-III so that the criterion standards used would be consistent with those used in current clinical practice. We limited the search to articles involving human subjects 18 years of age and older and published in the English language. We combined terms for the disorders with a validated search filter for retrieving articles on the diagnosis of health disorders.[23,24] Our final search terms included generalized anxiety disorder, panic disorder, questionnaires, screening, sensitivity, specificity, likelihood, medical history taking, and accuracy as well as terms for individual screening tools that were identified during our initial review of the search results (Appendix A).

We developed our search strategy in consultation with a master librarian. We supplemented electronic searching by examining the bibliographies of review articles, systematic reviews, and included studies. We also consulted experts in the field.

STUDY SELECTION

Using prespecified inclusion and exclusion criteria, two reviewers assessed titles and abstracts for relevance. Full-text articles, identified by either reviewer as potentially relevant, were retrieved for further review. Each article retrieved was examined by two reviewers against the eligibility criteria in Appendix B; disagreements were resolved by discussion or by a third reviewer. Studies excluded at the full-text review stage are listed with the reasons for exclusion in Appendix C.

Although KQ 1 was developed to focus on general medical patients with somatic symptoms, we chose to include studies with unselected patients presenting to general medical settings. We broadened the population criteria because few studies addressed only patients with specific somatic symptoms, and we reasoned that somatic symptoms were common (even if not specifically documented) in unselected general medical patients.[25] To identify studies most applicable to the Veteran population in the U.S., we included studies that examined measures in English or Spanish and were conducted in North America, Western Europe, New Zealand, or Australia. Detailed eligibility criteria are described in Table 1.

Table 1. Summary of inclusion and exclusion criteria

Study characteristic	Inclusion criteria	Exclusion criteria
Study design	Prospective comparison of an anxiety questionnaire to a reference standard	Case control studies that select patients with known disease and compare to healthy controls
Population	Adults ≥18 in general medical clinics with or without somatic symptoms.	Study populations of patients with preexisting mental health diagnosis
Instrument	Self-report instrument used to measure GAD or PD that is feasible to use in a medical setting without need for specialized equipment	Instruments requiring interviewer administration
Reference standard	Criteria based on DSM III or later; ICD 9 or later	Studies without an independent criterion standard
Outcome	Study reports a measure of sensitivity/specificity or data to derive an n*k table to validate operating characteristics.	Data to calculate sensitivity or specificity not provided
Setting	Primary care clinics including general internal medicine, family medicine and geriatrics; general medical and selected specialty medical settings (e.g., emergency departments, cardiology, gastrointestinal clinics, rheumatology and women's health)	Highly specialized clinics (e.g., memory disorder clinic) and psychiatric or mental health clinics

DATA ABSTRACTION

We abstracted data pertinent to the KQs into a data abstraction form (Appendix D). Key data included:

- study design
- setting
- population characteristics
- subject eligibility and exclusion criteria
- number of subjects
- details about the index test and criterion standard and their application
- psychiatric and medical comorbidities of the sample and outcomes

Data elements selected for abstraction were informed by the principles outlined by the Standards for Reporting of Diagnostic Accuracy (STARD).[26] These elements included descriptors to assess applicability (e.g., setting, sample characteristics, anxiety disorder prevalence) and quality elements (e.g., recruitment method, blinding, reference standard, sample size). When provided, raw data for the n*k table was abstracted, and when not provided, data were derived from other performance characteristics such as sensitivity and specificity.

We abstracted data for all relevant thresholds when data for more than one threshold of the index test were reported. If data were analyzed for subgroups based on race or sex, we abstracted them in separate n*k tables to address KQ 3. Performance characteristics such as sensitivity and specificity were recalculated by each investigator performing the abstraction to validate the data. When results were adjusted for the sampling design (e.g., partial verification of the criterion based diagnosis), we use the adjusted results.

All data abstractions were confirmed by a second reviewer. Disagreements were resolved by consensus or by obtaining a third reviewer's opinion when consensus could not be reached. Further, one author independently abstracted and validated all the n*k tables to check for accuracy.

QUALITY ASSESSMENT

We adopted a two-step approach to rate the quality of the evidence. First, we applied the Quality Assessment of Diagnostic Accuracy Studies (QUADAS) criteria for each study. QUADAS is a 14-item tool that was developed to assess the quality of diagnostic accuracy studies included in systematic reviews so that appropriate conclusions can be drawn in the context of potential biases.[27,28] Each item has three possible answers: Yes, No, and Unclear. The QUADAS criteria were applied for each study by the reviewer abstracting the article; this initial assessment was then overread by a second reviewer. Disagreements were resolved between the two reviewers, or when needed, by arbitration from a third reviewer.

To make QUADAS most relevant to studies of self-report tests for anxiety disorders, we modified question number 12 of the tool to ask: "Was the cutoff point for the test chosen a priori?" The rationale for this is many psychiatric scales intended for diagnostic purposes can have markedly different performance characteristics based on the cutoff used, with sensitivity and specificity changing in opposite directions. Not choosing the cutoff a priori, ideally based on prior research, can introduce bias and result in poor replicability in subsequent samples. The QUADAS criteria with our modification are detailed in Appendix E.

We then assigned a level of evidence for each study based on the elements covered in the QUADAS criteria. The levels of evidence ranged from I to V, with I being the highest level of evidence with a low risk of bias and V being the lowest level of evidence with a high risk for overestimating the accuracy of the test. The above assessment of quality is recommended by the Rational Clinical Exam series in the Journal of the American Medical Association (http://jama. ama-assn.org/cgi/collection/rational_clinical_exam). We also assessed studies for applicability to U.S. Veterans.

DATA SYNTHESIS

We critically analyzed studies to compare their characteristics, methods, and findings. Data derived from the studies for n*k tables were used to calculate performance measures (e.g., sensitivity, specificity) for each individual study. We then explored heterogeneity among the studies using Cochran's Q and the I^2, which describes the percentage of total variation across studies that is due to heterogeneity rather than to chance.[29] Heterogeneity was categorized as low, moderate, or high based on I^2 values of 25 percent, 50 percent, and 75 percent respectively. We also plotted study outcomes on a graph and visually evaluated the variation in study results. To further explore heterogeneity, we examined whether a threshold effect was present. A strong positive correlation between the sensitivities (and 1-specificities) is suggestive of a threshold effect. This is calculated as a Spearman correlation coefficient between the logit sensitivity and logit of 1-specificity. In the absence of a threshold effect, data were pooled, when statistically appropriate, using a random effects model. When a threshold effect was present, we analyzed the data using a summary receiver operating characteristic (ROC) curve.

Because GAD and PD are two distinct clinical entities, we did not attempt to combine the studies reporting on instruments that were specific to one or the other. Instead, we grouped them into two categories, studies on instruments specific for GAD and studies on instruments specific for PD, for analyses of heterogeneity. When an instrument was nonspecific and screened for both GAD and PD, we included it in both groups. When studies reported data to derive n*k tables by race or ethnicity, we calculated performance characteristics for each group for comparison.

Outliers were defined as studies that were markedly different from other included studies, due to either methodological or sample characteristics, or if they were significant outliers on visual inspection of forest plots of the operating characteristics. When we observed significant heterogeneity in operating characteristics, we recomputed summary estimates and test statistics after outliers were removed. Analysis was conducted using the open source software Meta-Disc, version 1.4 (Unit of Clinical Biostatistics, Ramón y Cajal Hospital, Madrid, Spain)[30]for all analyses except when we statistically combined data using a random effects model for which we used MetaAnalyst version Beta 3.13 (Tufts Medical Center).[31]

Because reading levels were not reported, we determined the reading level for each questionnaire using the Flesch-Kincaid Grade level readability formula through the corresponding Microsoft Word application.[32]

RATING THE BODY OF EVIDENCE

In addition to rating the quality of individual studies, we evaluated the overall quality of the evidence for each KQ as proposed by the GRADE Working Group.[33] In brief, the GRADE approach requires assessment of four domains: risk of bias, consistency, directness, and precision. Additional domains are to be used when appropriate. These domains were considered qualitatively, and two reviewers assigned a summary rating after discussion as High, Moderate, Low, or Insufficient strength of evidence according to the following criteria:

- High—Further research is very unlikely to change our confidence on the estimate of effect.

- Moderate—Further research is likely to have an important impact on our confidence in the estimate of effect and may change the estimate.

- Low—Further research is very likely to have an important impact on our confidence in the estimate of effect and is likely to change the estimate.

- Insufficient—Evidence on an outcome is absent or too weak, sparse, or inconsistent to estimate an effect.

In some cases, high, moderate, or low ratings were not possible or imprudent to make. In these situations, a grade of Insufficient was assigned.[33]

PEER REVIEW

A draft version of the report was reviewed by technical experts and clinical leadership, and their comments are provided in Appendix F.

RESULTS

LITERATURE FLOW

We identified 2890 unique citations from a combined electronic search of MEDLINE® via PubMed® (n = 982), PsycINFO® (n = 1472), and Cochrane Library (n = 413) and a manual examination of references (n = 23); zero additional articles were identified from an updated search of relevant systematic reviews. After applying inclusion and exclusion criteria, 2824 articles were excluded at the title-and-abstract level. We retrieved 66 articles for full-text review and excluded 54. For data abstraction and evidence synthesis, we retained a total of 12 articles representing 9 unique studies. Figure 2 illustrates each step of our literature search process.

Figure 2. Literature flow diagram

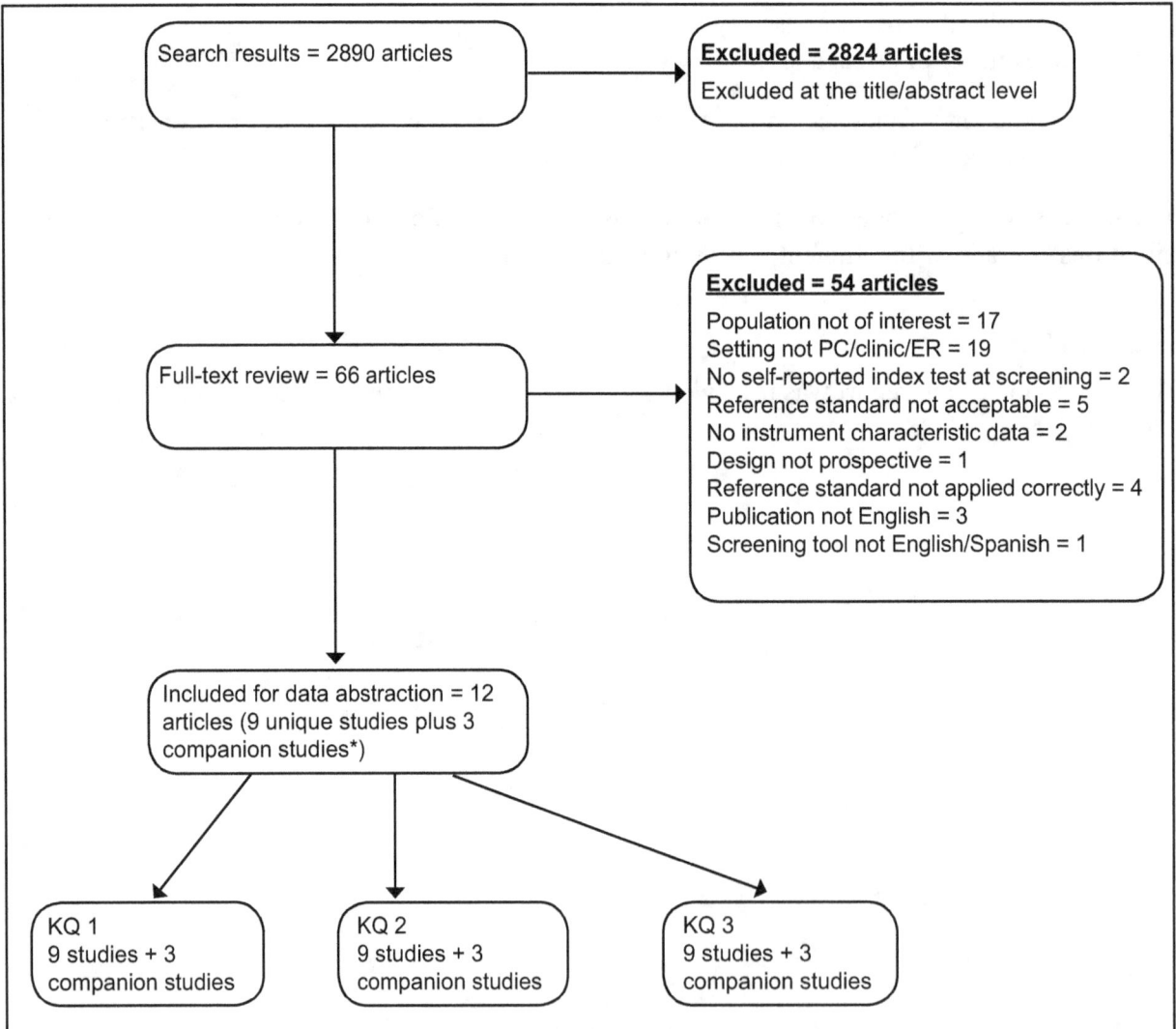

*Article reference list includes additional references cited for background and methods plus Web sites relevant to key questions. Companion studies are articles containing additional data pertinent to the unique, primary studies that were abstracted.

KQ 1. In general medical patients with somatic symptoms, what are the performance characteristics (e.g., sensitivity, specificity) of self-report questionnaires for diagnosing generalized anxiety disorder or panic disorder?

Self-report Measures

We identified nine studies that validated eight self-report measures of GAD and PD in primary care and general medical settings. Of these, two measures were GAD specific: Anxiety Disorder Scale–Generalized Anxiety and the Generalized Anxiety Disorder-7.[34,35] Three measures were PD specific: an unnamed 10-item questionnaire,[36] the Patient Health Questionnaire module for panic disorder,[18] and the Brief Panic Disorder Screen.[37] Two measures were multicomponent: Primary Care Evaluation of Mental Disorders[38] and Symptom Driven Diagnostic System–Primary Care.[39,40] One measure addressed both GAD and PD: Beck Anxiety Inventory–Primary Care.[41] All of the questionnaires were self-administered and did not require specialized equipment or trained personnel, making them suitable for patients to complete in a variety of settings.

Symptom Driven Diagnostic System-Primary Care (SDDS-PC)

The SDDS-PC is a two-stage instrument developed to diagnose mental disorders in primary care clinics. The first stage is a brief self-administered screen for six disorders including GAD and PD. Each positive screen requires further administration of a detailed diagnostic module. Among the instruments included in this review, the SDDS-PC is the only one that has been validated in more than one study; however, the versions tested in the two articles are slightly different. Leon and colleagues tested a 26-item scale with 4 items for GAD and 5 items for PD,[39] whereas Broadhead and colleagues tested an earlier version with 3 items for anxiety and 2 for GAD.[40]

Primary Care Evaluation of Mental Disorders (PRIME-MD)

The PRIME-MD was developed in the early 1990s to diagnose common mental illnesses, including anxiety disorders, in medical populations. It is a multicomponent questionnaire with two stages, the first of which is a brief screen consisting of 26 items, of which 3 address anxiety. If the patient answers yes to any of these questions, the physician is then prompted to use a diagnostic module for that disorder.[38] The two-step process takes 5 to 6 minutes in patients without a mental illness versus 11 to 12 minutes in those with a diagnosis. This was considered a barrier to use in routine clinical settings and subsequently led to the development of the Patient Health Questionnaire and Generalized Anxiety Disorder-7.

Patient Health Questionnaire (PHQ)

The PHQ is a three-page instrument that addresses depression, PD, other anxiety disorders, eating disorders, and alcohol abuse. After completion of the self-report form by the patient, the clinician can apply the abbreviated algorithm at the end of each page to make a diagnostic decision.[18] Though the PHQ specifically addresses PD, it is not specific to GAD.

Generalized Anxiety Disorder-7 (GAD-7)

The GAD-7 is a seven-item questionnaire specific to the diagnosis of GAD. It was developed to be a short instrument that can be used in primary care settings. An affirmative answer on any of the seven primary questions requires the patient to answer one more question about the effect of symptoms on functioning at work, home, and relationships. The authors suggested that, in addition to diagnosing GAD, this instrument could be used for tracking the severity of symptoms since cut points of 5, 10, and 15 could be interpreted as mild, moderate, and severe level of anxiety.[35]

Beck Anxiety Inventory-Primary Care (BAI-PC)

The BAI-PC is an abbreviated version of the more commonly known Beck Anxiety Inventory.[42] The seven items included in the BAI-PC are said to represent a "subjective dimension" of anxiety and include "unable to relax," "fear of the worst happening," "terrified," "nervous," "fear of losing control," "fear of dying," and "scared." The authors proposed that not including somatic symptoms might help screen out medical patients without anxiety and thereby increase the specificity of the instrument.

Anxiety Disorder Scale-Generalized Anxiety (ADS-GA)

The ADS-GA was developed as an instrument to detect anxiety disorders in individuals 65 years of age and older. The scale is an 11-item questionnaire in a dichotomous Yes/No format. Early validation studies determined the optimum cutoff to be 4 or 5 positive responses out of a possible 11 items.[43] Krasucki and colleagues validated this instrument in an outpatient geriatric population and developed a shortened version called the FEAR (frequency of anxiety; enduring nature of anxiety; alcohol or sedative use; restlessness or fidgeting). However, the shortened version has not been evaluated in an independent sample.[34]

Brief Panic Disorder Scale (BPDS)

The BPDS is a subscale of the 16-item Anxiety Sensitivity Inventory (ASI), a self-report measure used to assess sensitivity to the physical sensations associated with panic, such as heart racing and dizziness.[44] The subscale was derived in a sample of patients from an anxiety disorders clinic.[45] It consists of four items, all of which start with "It scares me when I …" and are followed by symptoms that include "feel shaky," "feel faint," "become short of breath," and "heart beats rapidly." Johnson and colleagues then validated this in a biracial primary care population.[37]

Unnamed 10-item questionnaire for PD

The 10-item instrument for the diagnosis of PD developed by Barsky and colleagues is unique in that it was derived in a sample of patients who were referred to an ambulatory electrocardiogram laboratory for the evaluation of palpitations. All of the other instruments were studied in unselected patients presenting to a general medical setting. The 10-item instrument was then validated in an independent sample of 124 patients referred for Holter monitoring of palpitations.[36] This scale has not been studied in other populations, and so the performance might vary based on patient characteristics.

Table 2 summarizes the characteristics of the 8 self-report measures.

Performance Characteristics of Self-report Instruments for Diagnosing Generalized Anxiety and Panic Disorders in Primary Care

Table 2. Characteristics of 8 self-report measures for GAD and PD

Instrument	Number of items	Scope	Response format	Timeframe	Score range	Usual cut point	Literacy levels[a]	Completion time	Tracking of symptoms
BAI-PC	7	GAD and PD	4 items of symptom severity	Past 2 weeks to today	0-21	≥ 5	Easy	≈ 1 minute[46]	Unknown
PRIME-MD	3	Multiple components with GAD and PD	Yes or No	Past month	0-3	≥ 1	Easy	<1 minute	No
SDDS-PC	5-PD	PD	Yes or No	Past month	0-5	Unclear	Easy	<2 minutes	Yes (scale has a separate longitudinal tracking module)
	4-GAD	GAD	Yes or No	6 months	0-5	Unclear	Easy	<2 minutes	
GAD-7	7	GAD	4 frequency ratings: "Not at all," "several days," "more than half the days," "nearly every day"	2 weeks	0-21	5 = mild 10 = moderate 15 = severe	Average	Unknown	Unknown
ADS-GA	11	GAD	Yes or No	Unknown	0-11	4–5	Easy	Unknown	Unknown
PHQ (panic module from original 3 page diagnostic form)	5 questions (5th has 11 subitems)	PD	Yes or No	4 weeks	0-5	Yes on first 4 questions with yes on 4 of the 11 subitems for question 5	Easy	< 1 for 42% 1 to 2 for 43% 3 to 5 for 13% > 5 for 3%	No
BPDS	4	PD	Symptom severity: "Very Little," "A Little," "Some," "Much," "Very Much"	None	0-16	≥ 11	Average	Unknown	Unknown
Unnamed scale	10	PD	Symptom severity: "not at all," "a little bit," "moderately," "quite a bit," "a great deal"	Unknown	0-50	> 21	Average	Unknown	Unknown

[a]Easy indicated third- to fifth-grade reading level; average, sixth- to ninth-grade reading level.[47]

15

Characteristics of Included Studies

Table 3 summarizes the characteristics of the nine studies included in this evidence synthesis. The sample sizes among the studies varied widely ranging from 56 to 3000. Other than one study that was conducted on patients attending a referral clinic for Holter monitoring,[36] all other studies were conducted in general medical clinics. One study selected patients presenting with palpitations;[36] all other studies recruited patients without regard to the presenting medical problem. None of the studies were conducted in VA hospitals or clinics; however, all but one of the studies were conducted in the U.S.

All of the studies had a high proportion of women ($\geq 60\%$), which might make the samples somewhat different from a predominantly male Veteran population. All but one study [34] reported the distribution of race, which was predominantly white but varied widely between studies (35 to 98%). In most of the studies, the screening instrument was self-administered. In one study in which 22 percent of the participants had not completed high school, a research assistant verbally administered the test to those who had difficulty reading.[48] Seven studies reported educational achievement among the participants, and the proportion of patients who had completed high school ranged from 77.8 to 94 percent.

Table 3. Characteristics of 9 included studies

Study	Setting and patient selection	Sample characteristics[a]	Prevalence	Instrument and threshold	Criterion standard	Quality rating
Beck et al., 1997[41]	Primary care Unselected	N: 56 Age: 48.54 (15.52) Female: 73%	GAD or PD: 23%	BAI-PC 5	DSM IIIR	III
Spitzer et al., 1994[38]	Primary care Unselected	N: 431 Age:55 (16.5) Female: 60%	GAD or PD: 17.9%	PRIME-MD $\geq$ 1	DSM IIIR	I
Broadhead et al.,1995(a)[40]	Primary care Unselected	N: 388 Age: 39.4 (12.4) Female: 72%	GAD: 3.09% PD: 6.9%	SDDS-PC	DSM IIIR	I
Broadhead et al.,1995(b)[40]	Primary care Unselected	N:257 Age: 40.3 (13.2) Female: 70%	GAD: 5.44% PD: 6.2%	SDDC-PC	DSM IIIR	I
Leon et al., 1996 [39]	Primary care Unselected	N: 501 Age: 49.4 Female: 66%	GAD: 15.96% PD: 7.9%	SDDC-PC	DSM IV	I
Spitzer et al., 1999[18]	Primary care Unselected	N: 585 Age: 46 (17.2) Female: 66%	PD: 7.0%	PHQ	DSM IIIR	I
Krasucki et al., 1999[34]	Primary care Unselected	N: 40 Age: 72.6 (NR) Female: 64%	GAD: 15.0%	ADS-GA	ICD 10	III
Barsky et al., 1997[36]	Specialty clinic Palpitations	N: 124 Age: 47.36 (NR) Female : 57%	PD: 25.8%	Un-named instrument	DSM IIIR	II
Spitzer et al., 2006[35]	Primary care Unselected	N: 965 Age: 47.4 (15.5) Female: 65%	GAD: 7.6%	GAD-7	DSM IV	I
Johnson et al., 2007[48]	Primary care Unselected	N: 295 Age: 54.1 (11.2) Female: 66%	PD: 13.9%	BPDS	DSM IV	I

[a]Reported Ns were calculated based on the number of patients who completed the criterion standard and not based on number enrolled in study.

Performance Characteristics of Self-report Measures

Table 4 shows performance characteristics of the self-report measures in the primary care setting (along with 95% confidence intervals). An ideal self-report measure has a high sensitivity (a high proportion of patients with an anxiety disorder have a positive self-report) and a high specificity (a high proportion of patients without an anxiety disorder have a negative self-report). Likelihood ratios are a measure of how useful the self-report is based on sensitivity and specificity. Values may range from 0 to infinity, with values above 1 increasing and values below 1 decreasing the likelihood of an anxiety disorder. The likelihood ratio positive indicates how much more likely a positive self-report comes from a patient with, rather than without, an anxiety disorder. The likelihood ratio negative indicates how much more likely a negative self-report comes from a patient with, rather than without, an anxiety disorder. When coupled with the pretest probability of disease, the likelihood ratio allows ready calculation of posttest probability of disease. In general, diagnostic tests with likelihood ratios ≥ 5 or ≤ 0.2 have large effects on the posttest probability of disease.

Table 4. Performance characteristics of self-report measures in primary care settings

Study	Instrument	Sensitivity	Specificity	Likelihood ratio positive	Likelihood ratio negative
GAD and PD					
Spitzer et al., 1994[38]	PRIME-MD	0.93 (0.85 to 0.98)	0.53 (0.48 to 0.58)	1.99 (1.76 to 2.26)	0.12 (0.05 to 0.29)
Beck et al, 1997[41]	BAI-PC	0.85 (0.55 to 0.98)	0.81 (0.67 to 0.92)	4.55 (2.33 to 8.86)	0.19 (0.05 to 0.68)
GAD specific					
Broadhead et al., 1995(a)[40]	SDDS-PC	0.92 (0.61 to 1.00)	0.54 (0.49 to 0.59)	1.99 (1.63 to 2.44)	0.15 (0.02 to 1.01)
Broadhead et al., 1995(b)[40]	SDDS-PC	0.86 (0.57 to 0.98)	0.60 (0.53 to 0.66)	2.12 (1.63 to 2.76)	1.12 (1.63 to 2.76)
Leon et al., 1996[39]	SDDS-PC	0.74 (0.63 to 0.83)	0.82 (0.78 to 0.85)	4.08 (3.21 to 5.20)	0.32 (0.22 to 0.46)
Krasucki et al., 1999[34]	ADS-GA	0.40 (0.05 to 0.85)	0.86 (0.70-0.95)	2.88 (0.75 to 11.07)	0.70 (0.34 to 0.46)
Spitzer et al., 2006[35]	GAD-7	0.89 (0.79 to 0.95)	0.82 (0.79 to 0.84)	4.93 (4.20 to 5.80)	0.13 (0.07 to 0.26)
PD specific					
Spitzer et al., 1999[18]	PHQ	0.80 (0.65 to 0.91)	0.99 (0.98 to 1.00)	87.41 (36.06 to 211.88)	0.20 (0.11 to 0.37)
Broadhead et al., 1995(a)[40]	SDDS-PC	0.78 (0.58 to 0.91)	0.80 (0.76 to 0.84)	3.90 (2.92 to 5.20)	0.28 (0.14 to 0.56)
Broadhead et al., 1995(b)[40]	SDDS-PC	0.62 (0.35 to 0.85)	0.83 (0.78 to 0.88)	3.77 (2.34 to 6.05)	0.45 (0.24 to 0.85)
Leon et al., 1996[39]	SDDS-PC	0.70 (0.53 to 0.83)	0.91 (0.88 to 0.93)	7.87 (5.51 to 11.23)	0.33 (0.20 to 0.53)
Barsky et al., 1997[36]	10-item scale	0.72 (0.53 to 0.86)	0.71 (0.60 to 0.80)	2.45 (1.67 to 3.60)	0.40 (0.22 to 0.70)
Johnson et al., 2007[48]	BPDS	0.61 (0.44 to 0.76)	0.29 (0.23 to 0.35)	0.86 (0.66 to 1.11)	1.36 (0.88 to 2.08)

The PRIME-MD had a relatively high sensitivity compared to its specificity, which is not surprising given that the screen has three broad questions intended to prompt further physician interview. Among the instruments that screen for GAD, the GAD-7 had good sensitivity and specificity with comparable likelihood ratios. However, this instrument has been validated in only one population.

The SDDS-PC has been validated in more than one population; however, the versions in the two studies are slightly different in that the study by Broadhead and colleagues[40] tested the 16-item SDDS-PC with 2 questions for GAD and 3 for PD corresponding to the DSM-IIIR, whereas the study by Leon and colleagues[39] tested a 26-item instrument under the same name with 4 questions for GAD and 5 for PD made to correspond to DSM-IV. Not surprisingly, the SDDS-PC showed variable performance characteristics depending on the version and the sample. The two samples (initial validation and cross validation) in the study by Broadhead and colleagues[40] were significantly different in race, education, and marital status.

The ADS-GA was unique in that it was the only study conducted outside the U.S., and the population in the study was also substantially older, with a mean age of 72.6 years. The ADS-GA had low sensitivity (40%) for GAD, making its performance and study population an outlier in this group of studies.

Among the studies that examined instruments specific for panic disorder, the PHQ had the highest sensitivity and specificity with a very high positive predictive value and a moderately good negative predictive value. Other instruments, the BAI-PC, the 10-item scale, and the BPDS are not discussed further due to very small sample sizes and/or unimpressive performance characteristics.

Examination of Heterogeneity and Statistical Pooling of Data

Because GAD and PD are two distinct illnesses with unique courses and differences in response to treatment, we did not attempt to statistically combine the studies; instead, we analyzed them in two groups: GAD-specific instruments and PD-specific instruments. However, for analysis purposes, we did combine the two studies that screened for both GAD and PD[38,41] with both groups. We also conducted a sensitivity analysis without the above two studies to determine if they contributed significantly to heterogeneity.

For GAD, the test for heterogeneity (Cochran's Q) was statistically significant ($p<0.001$) for all 4 performance characteristics (sensitivity, specificity, positive predictive value, and negative predictive value). The I^2 ranged from 78.3 to 97.2 percent, which indicated a high level of heterogeneity. Sensitivity analysis without the two nonspecific instruments did not significantly decrease the heterogeneity. Neither did repeating the analysis without the study by Krasucki and colleagues,[34] which, on visual inspection of plots, appeared to be an outlier.

To further explore heterogeneity, we examined if a threshold effect was present. The Spearman correlation coefficient between the logit sensitivity and logit of 1-specificity was 0.786 ($p = 0.036$), which suggests a threshold effect. A threshold effect can occur when different studies examining an instrument use different thresholds for diagnosis, resulting in varying sensitivities and specificities. However, it is unlikely here since the studies included were examining different instruments, which in itself can contribute to heterogeneity. Further, partial verification bias and differences in samples and settings can also contribute to heterogeneity. In this analysis, all studies were conducted with unselected patients from primary care settings, but diagnostic standards and assessment methods varied across studies, which could have contributed to a threshold effect.

For PD, the test for heterogeneity (Cochran's Q) was statistically significant (p<0.001) and I^2 ranged from 71.4 to 99.0 percent, again indicating a high level of heterogeneity. Sensitivity analyses without the nonspecific instruments did not significantly reduce heterogeneity. We again explored the presence of a threshold effect, but in this case, the Spearman correlation coefficient was –0.071 ($p = 0.867$), indicating that a threshold effect is unlikely to contribute to heterogeneity. Because the patients in the study by Barsky and colleagues[36] were significantly different in that they were all referred for Holter monitoring of palpitations and had a high prevalence of PD, we conducted a sensitivity analysis without this study but did not find a change in the heterogeneity. Given the high degree of heterogeneity, we did not statistically combine the results from the all studies to yield summary estimates of sensitivity and specificity. Instead, we plotted the results on a summary receiver operating characteristic curve (SROC) for each disorder (Figures 3 and 4). A summary ROC displays the trade-off between sensitivity and specificity. Several useful statistical properties are reported in the figures, including the area under the curve (AUC) and the Q*. The AUC is a measure of the questionnaire's ability to discriminate between those with and without an anxiety disorder. A value of 0.5 is no better than chance, while a value of 1.0 represents perfect diagnostic test discrimination; tests with values greater than 0.80 are generally considered to have good discriminate properties. The Q* statistic is the point on the SROC where sensitivity equals specificity. As can be seen in Figures 3 and 4, the questionnaires collectively have good overall test performance.

Figure 3. SROC curve for GAD measures

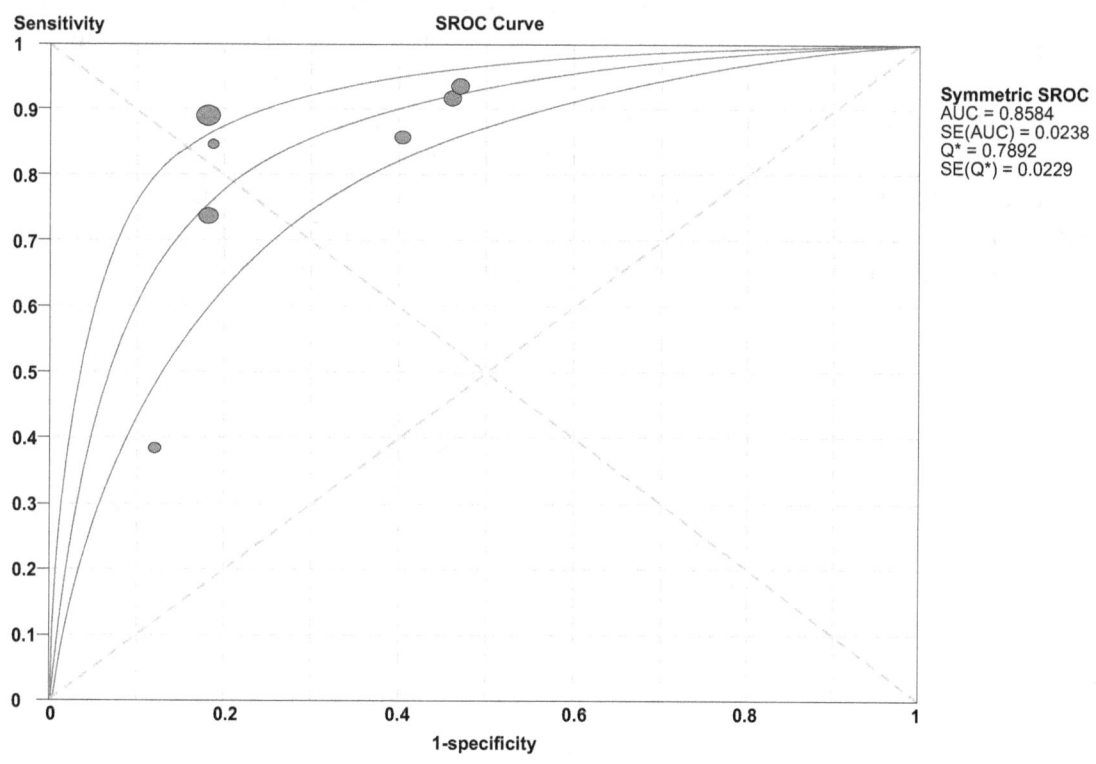

Figure 4. SROC curve for PD measures

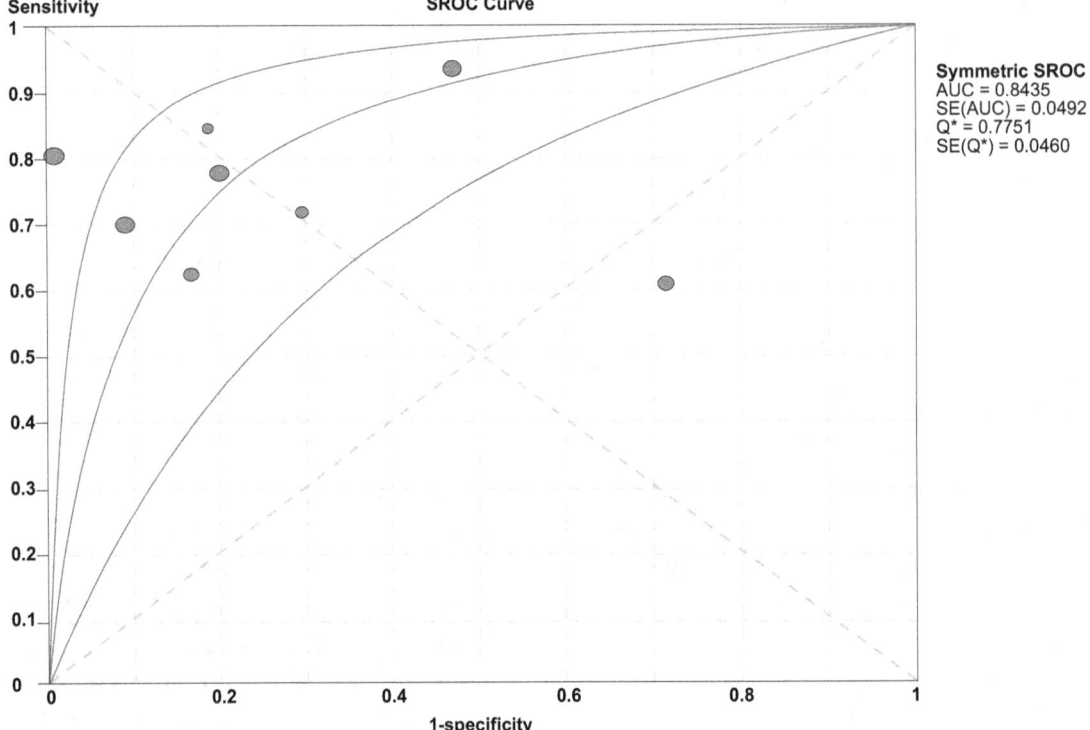

We did an exploratory analysis of the three studies that validated the SDDS-PC. Heterogeneity for GAD was moderate to high, and there was a high threshold effect with a Spearman correlation coefficient of 1 ($p < 0.001$). However, for PD, the heterogeneity was minimal for sensitivity (Cochran's Q = 1.19, df = 2, p = 0.55; I^2 of 0). Similarly, the heterogeneity for the negative likelihood ratio was also low (Cochran's Q = 1.09, df=2, p = 0.58; I^2 = 0). Heterogeneity for other operating characteristics was high. Overall threshold effect was small, with the Spearman correlation coefficient of 0.5 ($p = 0.67$). Therefore, we statistically combined the results for sensitivity and negative likelihood ratio of the SDDC-PC for PD using a random effects model. The pooled sensitivity for the SDDS-PC was 0.71 (95% CI 0.60 to 0.80) and the pooled negative likelihood ratio was 0.35 (95% CI 0.25 to 0.48) (Figure 5).

Figure 5. Forest plot of pooled sensitivity for studies that tested the SDDS-PC for PD

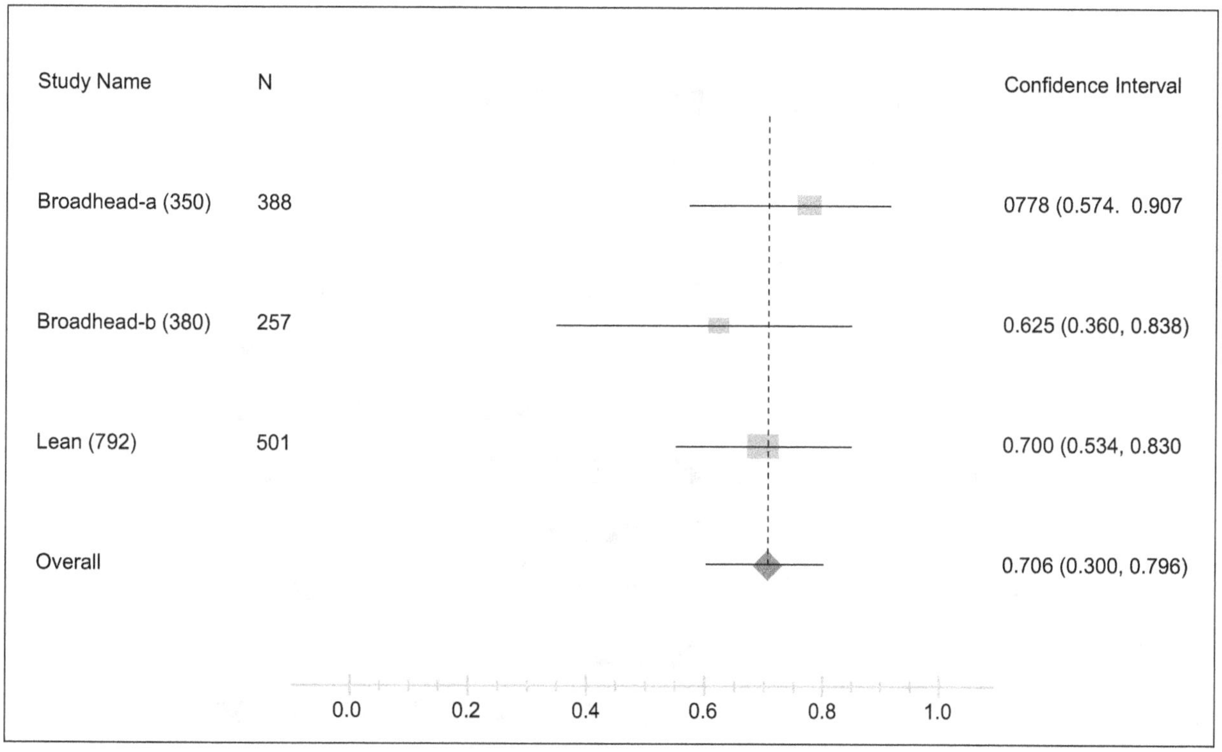

Study Name	N		Confidence Interval
Broadhead-a (350)	388		0778 (0.574. 0.907
Broadhead-b (380)	257		0.625 (0.360, 0.838)
Lean (792)	501		0.700 (0.534, 0.830
Overall			0.706 (0.300, 0.796)

Quality of Evidence for KQ 1

The quality of evidence for each of the studies was evaluated using the modified QUADAS. A summary graph of the quality is provided in Figure 6. All included studies gave clearly described inclusion criteria for patients, used accurate reference standards, and conducted the reference standard within a reasonable time. The study authors decided that administering the reference standard within a month of the index test would not affect the validity given that both PD and GAD exist for longer periods of time.

Most studies did not choose a cutoff a priori since many studies combined both the development and the validation of the scale—thus there was no established cutoff the investigators could use. This is a weakness because many of these validation studies have not been replicated. Also, many of the studies did not confirm the diagnosis using the reference standard in all, or in a random sample, of the patients, which could have contributed to partial verification bias.

Figure 6. QUADAS summaries for KQ 1

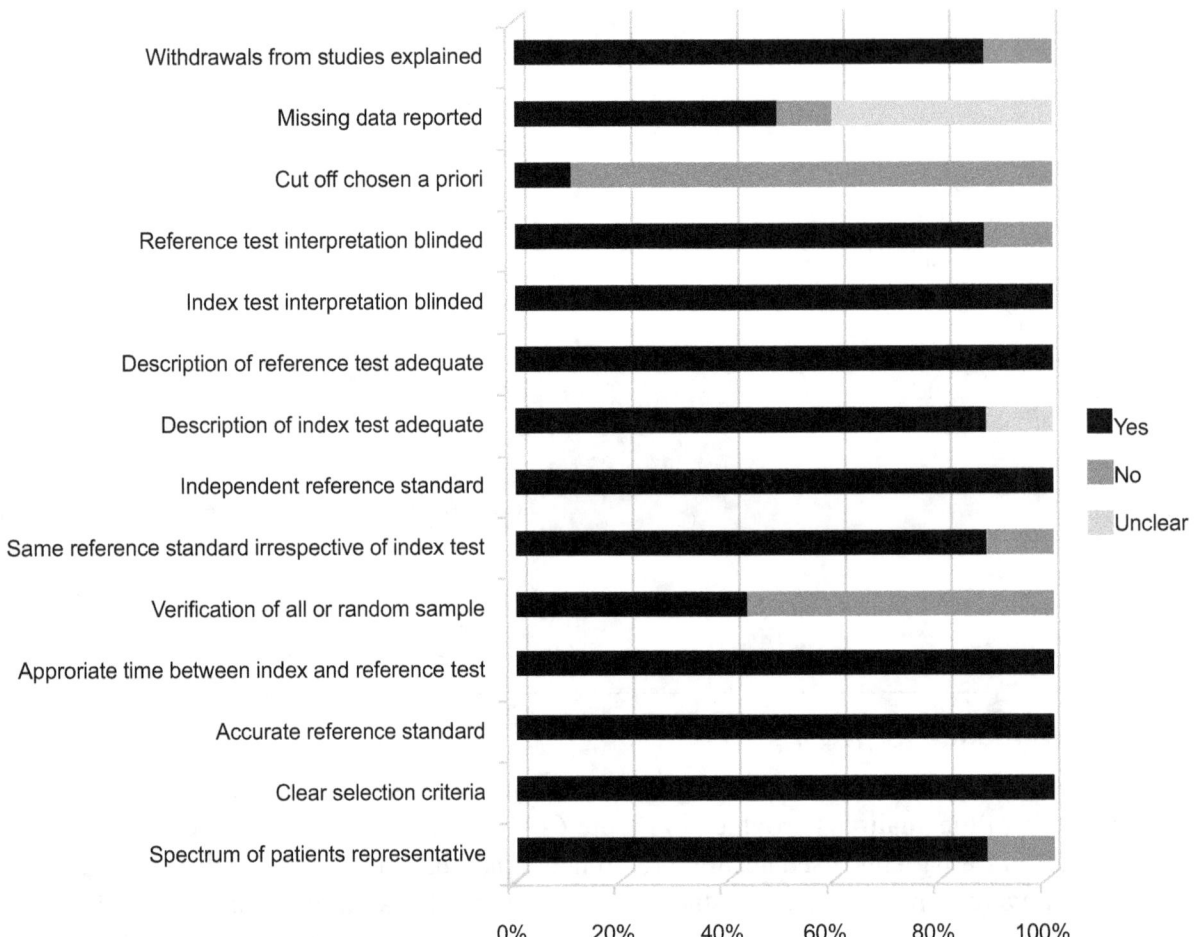

KQ 2. For questionnaires evaluated in KQ 1, which measures are most feasible to use in primary care settings? Specifically, what is the reading comprehension level, time required to complete, response format, and compatibility with telephone administration?

Studies of Efficacy

Based on considerations of feasibility, there is limited evidence to recommend one screening tool over another. Instrument characteristics regarding feasibility are summarized in Table 2. Most of the instruments are brief, with the number of questions ranging from 3 to 11. The GAD-7, BPDS, and 10-item PD instrument are at an average reading level (sixth to ninth grade), and the rest are at an easy reading level (third to fifth grade). The PRIME-MD has been validated for telephone administration and includes screening and diagnostic assessments for multiple common mental illnesses; the 3-item screening measure for anxiety disorders takes less than 1 minute to complete.[49] The average time taken to complete all sections of the PRIME-MD diagnostic interview, triggered by positive responses on the associated screening component, was 8.4 minutes, which in a busy clinic was found to be too high to be practical.[38] The following observations are about selected instruments that may be promising based on our qualitative assessment of their feasibility.

For PD, the panic module of the PHQ is a short, self-report instrument with reading and comprehension at the third- to fifth-grade level and a simple yes/no response format. In the initial validation study, 42 percent of patients took less than 1 minute to complete the questionnaire, 43 percent took 2 to 3 minutes, and 13 percent took more than 5 minutes. We did not identify any studies where the feasibility of telephone administration of the PHQ was studied. However, both the yes/no and the 4-item Likert response formats of the PHQ for depression have been used successfully with telephone administration.[50] Considering feasibility as a function of performance of the instrument, in an average primary care clinic with a 7 percent prevalence of PD, a clinician seeing 100 patients per week can expect 6 to 7 patients to screen positive for PD, while 1 patient might not be identified by the instrument. Of patients who screen positive, almost all will have PD. One disadvantage is that the PHQ panic module, unlike the PHQ-9 for depression, has been studied rigorously in only one large sample.[18]

For generalized anxiety disorder, the GAD-7 is a short, well-performing instrument that assesses the severity of DSM -IV criteria symptoms over the past 2 weeks. Unlike the dichotomized response format of the panic module of the PHQ, the GAD-7 has four response options reflecting increased levels of severity. Both the 2-week time period and the graded response format might be useful in tracking response to treatment; however, responsiveness has not been studied formally. In a primary care clinic with GAD prevalence of 7.6 percent, 23 out of 100 patients will screen positive for GAD, while 1 patient with GAD might not be identified by the instrument. Of patients who screen positive, 16 to 17 will not have GAD after a diagnostic evaluation (false positives) and 6 to 7 will be true positives. Similar to the PHQ for panic, the GAD-7 has been validated with a diagnostic standard in only one sample.[35]

The SDDS-PC has the advantage of being a single instrument for both GAD and PD along with other mental disorders, which can be useful in a busy primary care setting. However, the combined sensitivity of the instrument is lower than the GAD-7 and PHQ. Further, the SDDS then requires confirmation through a nurse-administered computer module that is entered using the SDDS-PC software. No recent studies of the SDDS-PC have been published, and it is uncertain if the needed software has been updated for modern computer operating systems. We did not identify any studies that examined its compatibility with telephone administration.

Quality of Evidence for KQ 2

We did not find studies that directly addressed the feasibility of the administration of the various instruments included in this review. Our assessment is based on the primary validation studies for KQ 1, discussed previously. Further, the assessment of reading level was not provided in the primary studies but was assessed by the authors using computer software.

KQ 3. For questionnaires evaluated in KQ 1, do the performance characteristics vary by gender, race, age group, or setting?

Among the self-report measures evaluated, none of the GAD studies and only one PD study reported a subgroup analysis. Johnson and colleagues[48] compared Caucasian to African-American patients, while no studies reported subgroup analyses by gender, age group, or setting for PD. The absence of such data suggests that additional research is needed to determine if the various screening measures perform similarly among different subpopulations.

The report by Johnson and colleagues[48] was good quality and differed from other studies only in the fact that the screening instrument was administered verbally to an unspecified number of participants who had difficulty reading. In the subgroup analysis, the study by Johnson and colleagues[48] compared the performance characteristics of the BPDS for 216 Caucasian versus 79 African-American primary care patients. Sensitivity data indicated that the questionnaire performed similarly in the two groups (Caucasian = .60, African American = .63, $\chi^2[1, N = 295] = 0.03$, p = .87). The questionnaire's specificity, however, significantly differed between the two groups (Caucasian = .25, African American = .60, $\chi^2[1, N = 295] = 0.75$, p = .03). These results indicate that the BPDS performed better among Caucasians because at the optimal cutoff of 10, there were more false positives among African Americans. Table 4 displays the sensitivity, specificity, positive likelihood ratio, and negative likelihood ratio from this study.

Qualitatively, there were differences in sensitivity and specificity among the two samples in the initial validation and cross-validation samples in the study by Broadhead and colleagues, which had different ethnic distributions.[40] The instrument, methods and quality of the two studies were the same. The initial validation sample was 97.9 percent white and 0.3 percent black, while the cross-validation sample had 71.9 percent white and 26 percent black ($p < 0.001$). The sensitivity and specificity were 0.92, 0.54 and 0.86, 0.60 respectively. However, the two samples also varied significantly in terms of education and marital status; therefore, one cannot conclude that the differences are exclusively due to the racial distribution.

SUMMARY AND DISCUSSION

Most of the instruments included in this review have moderate to good operating characteristics for the detection of GAD and PD in unselected primary care settings. Only one study specifically addressed test performance in a sample presenting with somatic symptoms, while the others assessed test performance on all patients presenting to primary care settings. Most of the instruments included in this review appear feasible for use in primary care based on comprehension level. However, it is uncertain if these instruments are responsive to change in symptom status and the specific values associated with a clinically important response are unknown. There is preliminary evidence from one study that test performance can vary based on race. There is a current lack of evidence about differences in test performance based on gender and setting.

SUMMARY OF EVIDENCE BY KEY QUESTION

A summary of the strength of evidence (SOE) for each KQ is in Table 5.

Table 5. Summary of strength of evidence by KQ

Number of studies (subjects)	Study quality	Consistency	Directness	Precision	SOE key finding
KQ 1: Performance characteristics in unselected primary care patients					
GAD					
6 (2638)	Good	Inconsistent (high heterogeneity)	Indirect	Imprecise	Moderate
PD					
7 (2513)	Good	Inconsistent (high heterogeneity)	Indirect	Imprecise	Moderate
KQ 2: Feasibility for use in primary care settings				SOE not formally assessed	
9(3518)	Good	Not applicable	Not applicable	Not applicable	
KQ 3: Variable performance by race					Low
1 (295)	Good	Not applicable	Direct	Sensitivity imprecise; specificity precise	Equivalent sensitivity but lower specificity in African Americans
KQ 3: Variable performance by gender, age, and setting					Insufficient
None	Not applicable	Not applicable	Not applicable	Not applicable	No studies

Our search identified a large number of anxiety measures, but few measures had been studied in primary care populations. These measures had moderate to good operating characteristics, but unlike instruments used in the detection of other common mental illnesses such as depression or dementia, the operating characteristics have not been replicated in multiple samples. Even for the SDDS-PC—the only instrument evaluated in multiple studies—the versions studied were different, which might change the test performance. Based on operating characteristics, we did not find sufficient evidence to recommend a single validated self-report measure in the screening of GAD or PD in primary care. Our results are congruent with the recent guidelines from the National Institute for Health and Clinical Excellence on GAD and PD.[51] However, based on study quality, operating characteristics, precision of the estimates, potential for assessing response to change, and other feasibility issues, the most promising instruments are: the panic module of the PHQ, the GAD-7 and the SDDS-PC.

It is important to note that all of the instruments included in this review are for screening or case-finding purposes and do not by themselves make a diagnosis of GAD and PD. A diagnosis must be established through further evaluation by a primary care physician or by a mental health professional to whom a patient is referred. All but one of the instruments were validated by screening unselected primary care patients. Therefore, it is possible that they might perform differently if the instrument is used for case-finding in a high-risk population. For example, patients who present with unexplained GI symptoms might have a higher incidence or severity of anxiety disorders and, therefore, change the performance of the instrument. We did not identify any studies that validated instruments in a case-finding situation except for the unnamed 10-item instrument by Barsky and colleagues.[36]

While the studies included in the review provide information about the performance of various screening instruments, the impact of screening for GAD and PD on direct, patient-related outcomes is not known. In the absence of direct evidence on the impact of screening for anxiety, we considered a number of theoretical implications. These included patients who receive a true negative test result might be reassured that they do not have a mental illness, and if they present with a physical symptom, medical causes for this might be investigated further. For those who receive a false positive test result, there might be distress from an incorrect diagnosis, a greater likelihood of receiving ineffective treatment, or a delay in diagnosis of the true cause of their symptoms. Patients who receive a false negative test result might continue to remain anxious due to a delay in effective treatment and might undergo unnecessary diagnostic testing in a futile search for other medical causes for the anxiety symptoms.

Though many of the above considerations are inferred rather than proven in studies, there is good evidence that anxiety disorders are underrecognized and that there are effective treatments for anxiety disorders, and thus screening has the potential to improve patient outcomes. One review of antidepressant medications found that the number needed to treat for GAD was 5.15 and that antidepressants were significantly better that placebo.[21] Similarly, various types of psychotherapy, including cognitive behavioral therapy and supportive therapy, have been shown to be better than treatment as usual for GAD.[52] Both tricyclic antidepressants and selective serotonin reuptake inhibitors (SSRIs) have been shown to be superior to placebo in the treatment of PD.[53] The mean effect size for acute treatment outcome for SSRIs relative to placebo was 0.55 (a moderate effect) in one analysis of twelve randomized controlled trials.[54] Psychotherapy as well as Internet-based therapy have been shown to be effective in treating PD.[55,56] Although not a test of anxiety screening per se, at least two care management trials have shown that screening, coupled with effective primary care treatment, improves clinical outcomes for patients with a variety of anxiety disorders.[16,20]

When evaluating screening instruments for anxiety, it is important to consider that the criteria for GAD will change with the new DSM-V. While still not final, one proposed change is to reduce the duration of symptoms of GAD from 6 to 3 months.[57] In the primary validation study for the GAD-7, 67 percent of patients with scores greater than 10 (the proposed cut point) had symptoms for more than 6 months, and 96 percent had symptoms more than 1 month.[35] With changes such as those mentioned above, the number of false positive results could decrease—but the number of false negatives would likely increase as the spectrum of disease is shifted to less chronic and potentially milder disease. Another proposed change is the addition of criterion D, which requires the presence of at least one of four avoidance behaviors that are not included in screening instruments based on DSM-III and DSM-IV editions. Thus, the implications on the performance characteristics of the current instruments are yet unknown.

In summary, the U.S. Preventive Services Task Force has not issued a recommendation on screening for anxiety disorders. Our review shows several promising self-report instruments that could be used in VA for case-finding or evaluated in studies to determine the impact of systematic screening. Currently, the best clinical use of these measures in primary care would be for case-finding in patients with somatic symptoms or other factors that heighten the suspicion of an anxiety disorder. The reorganization of VA primary care services into Patient Aligned Care Teams (PACTs) that better integrate mental health services may present an opportunity to test the utility of anxiety screening measures that are coupled with high-quality diagnostic evaluation and treatment.

STRENGTHS AND LIMITATIONS

An important limitation of the current review is the lack of studies reporting on patient outcomes and societal impact. This has been recognized as a challenge in systematic reviews of diagnostic tests.[58] We were unable to assess for publication bias because there is currently no reliable way to make this assessment for studies of diagnostic tests. Unlike studies of interventions, studies of diagnostic accuracy do not have a database such as ClinicalTrials.gov, where one can identify studies that were started but not published or which are ongoing—making the assessment of publication bias challenging.

The studies included in this report were heterogeneous and thus prevented the statistical pooling of data. Further, the number of studies identified was small and therefore limited our ability to do subgroup analyses or meta-regressions to further explain observed heterogeneity.

Our eligibility criteria were designed to exclude poor-quality studies (e.g., studies where the same person conducted the screening and criterion standard were excluded). As a result, all studies were of at least moderate quality. This means that some poor-quality studies that could provide low-level evidence on the topic might have been excluded from the review. However, we think that the solution to this would be to encourage high-quality validation studies.

We also excluded studies of instruments in languages other than English and Spanish as well as articles that were published in languages other than English. While this might have excluded studies that were otherwise rigorous in methodology, we thought that these studies would not be directly applicable to the U.S. Veteran population and therefore not relevant for this report.[59]

Despite these limitations, this report was a highly structured and systematic review of the extant evidence. Our evidence synthesis was guided by a carefully designed standardized protocol, including a systematic search of research databases and relevant bibliographies, double data abstraction, and use of validated criteria to assess the quality of identified studies. Our multidisciplinary team included expertise in internal medicine, primary care, psychiatry, and psychology.

RECOMMENDATIONS FOR FUTURE RESEARCH

Replication of the results for instruments with promising characteristics is needed to verify initial findings. Specifically, rigorous validation of these instruments in the VHA is needed to ascertain applicability to the Veteran population. Given the limited number of measures evaluated in primary care populations, some investigators might reasonably develop and test novel anxiety instruments. An important consideration for such an undertaking is whether to develop general screens for significant anxiety symptoms, or more specific measures that are disease specific. Disease-specific measures that screen for a range of disorders would likely require more items and take longer to complete than general measures but could facilitate diagnostic evaluation and better treatment matching. General and disease-specific measures may also differ in responsiveness to change. Whether general or disease specific, these instruments would be tested ideally in unselected primary care populations, in patients presenting with symptoms commonly associated with anxiety disorders (e.g., chest pain or insomnia), and in patients with common mental illnesses (e.g., depressive disorder) as a screen for a co-occurring anxiety disorder. Further, given the preliminary data suggesting a possible difference by race, these studies should be powered for subgroup differences. The presence of a higher proportion of older adults in the Veteran population is another reason for validation of these instruments in the VHA since detection of anxiety disorders among older adults is known to be especially challenging.[60]

To evaluate the effects of screening for anxiety disorders, RCTs would be needed that include important patient outcomes such as effects on symptom status and patient functioning. Given the lack of benefit from screening for depression as a single intervention, and the high likelihood of similar findings for anxiety disorders, these trials would need to include a structured treatment component. There are no current recommendations for routine screening of primary care patients with anxiety disorders though prevalence is high and there are demonstrable impacts on functioning. Establishing patient outcomes, such as the percentage of patients who go on to receive treatment, their quality of life, and treatment side effects, would be important in determining if screening for anxiety in primary care has an overall positive impact to the individual patient and to the health system and society at large. Alternatively, if RCTs are considered not practical, a formal process—such as one suggested by the U.S. Preventive Services Task Force that evaluates and links evidence from screening and treatment studies— could be used to evaluate the potential benefits of systematic screening.

Another consideration for future studies is the inclusion of feasibility questions in the study design that assess the feasibility of the instrument in an average clinic. Specifically, patient receptiveness to completing screening, time taken, incompletion rates, and validity of instruments when administered by telephone, handheld device, or Web compared with in-person screening are all critical to the comprehensive assessment of the effectiveness of an instrument. Responsiveness to change is another desirable characteristic and has been a key feature in the adoption of the PHQ-9 for depression. A similar evaluation of this property for anxiety instruments could promote uptake of these instruments into routine practice.

Summary of Recommendations

- Though none of the included scales have sufficient evidence to be recommended as the single best option, the PHQ, GAD-7, and SDDS-PC are the most promising based on performance and applicability. Future research should focus on replicating early findings.

- These scales should be considered for incorporation into the VA Mental Health Assistant to facilitate use by providers.

- The Primary Care–Mental Health Integration Program and PACT should consider anxiety measures that have the most evidence based on this review.

- VA Research and Development should consider supporting studies to evaluate the performance of these instruments in the Veteran population since performance may differ in older adults with high rates of medical and psychiatric comorbidities.

- The instruments should be evaluated for sensitivity to change to enable monitoring of illness and response to treatment.

- Studies should include assessments of the feasibility and validity of different modes of administration and should be powered to detect differences in the performance of instruments based on age, race, setting or ethnicity.

CONCLUSIONS

In summary, there are several promising case-finding instruments with good performance for GAD and PD in primary care populations. However, there has been little replication of initial validation studies. There is also a lack of evidence about the feasibility of these instruments for telephone administration and their sensitivity to change. Though there is preliminary evidence that test performance can vary by race, this has not been addressed by any of the major validation studies, and there have been no followup studies on this question. Studies are needed that replicate initial findings and systematically study feasibility and variations in performance based on race, gender, and setting.

REFERENCES

1. Hoffman DL, Dukes EM, Wittchen HU. Human and economic burden of generalized anxiety disorder. *Depress Anxiety*. 2008;25(1):72-90.

2. Schonfeld WH, Verboncoeur CJ, Fifer SK, et al. The functioning and well-being of patients with unrecognized anxiety disorders and major depressive disorder. *J Affect Disord*. 1997;43(2):105-19.

3. American Psychiatric Association Task Force on DSM-IV. *Diagnostic and statistical manual of mental disorders: DSM-IV-TR*. 4th ed Washington, DC: American Psychiatric Association; 2000.

4. Wittchen HU, Zhao S, Kessler RC, et al. DSM-III-R generalized anxiety disorder in the National Comorbidity Survey. *Arch Gen Psychiatry*. 1994;51(5):355-64.

5. Kessler RC, McGonagle KA, Zhao S, et al. Lifetime and 12-month prevalence of DSM-III-R psychiatric disorders in the United States. Results from the National Comorbidity Survey. *Arch Gen Psychiatry*. 1994;51(1):8-19.

6. Byers AL, Yaffe K, Covinsky KE, et al. High occurrence of mood and anxiety disorders among older adults: The National Comorbidity Survey Replication. *Arch Gen Psychiatry*. 2010;67(5):489-96.

7. Kroenke K, Spitzer RL, Williams JB, et al. Anxiety disorders in primary care: prevalence, impairment, comorbidity, and detection. *Ann Intern Med*. 2007;146(5):317-25.

8. Adler DA, Possemato K, Mavandadi S, et al. Psychiatric status and work performance of veterans of Operations Enduring Freedom and Iraqi Freedom. *Psychiatr Serv*. 2011;62(1):39-46.

9. Hoge CW, Castro CA, Messer SC, et al. Combat duty in Iraq and Afghanistan, mental health problems, and barriers to care. *N Engl J Med*. 2004;351(1):13-22.

10. Bridges KW, Goldberg DP. Somatic presentation of DSM III psychiatric disorders in primary care. *J Psychosom Res*. 1985;29(6):563-9.

11. Kirmayer LJ, Robbins JM, Dworkind M, et al. Somatization and the recognition of depression and anxiety in primary care. *Am J Psychiatry*. 1993;150(5):734-41.

12. Tyrer P, Baldwin D. Generalised anxiety disorder. *Lancet*. 2006;368(9553):2156-66.

13. Nutting PA, Rost K, Dickinson M, et al. Barriers to initiating depression treatment in primary care practice. *J Gen Intern Med*. 2002;17(2):103-11.

14. Rost K, Nutting P, Smith J, et al. The role of competing demands in the treatment provided primary care patients with major depression. *Arch Fam Med*. 2000;9(2):150-4.

15. Rubenstein LV, Williams JW, Jr., Danz M, et al. 2009.

16. Roy-Byrne P, Craske MG, Sullivan G, et al. Delivery of evidence-based treatment for multiple anxiety disorders in primary care: a randomized controlled trial. *JAMA*. 2010;303(19):1921-8.

17. Williams JW, Jr., Gerrity M, Holsinger T, et al. Systematic review of multifaceted interventions to improve depression care. *Gen Hosp Psychiatry*. 2007;29(2):91-116.

18. Spitzer RL, Kroenke K, Williams JB. Validation and utility of a self-report version of PRIME-MD: the PHQ primary care study. Primary Care Evaluation of Mental Disorders. Patient Health Questionnaire. *JAMA*. 1999;282(18):1737-44.

19. World Health Organization. AUDIT. The Alcohol Use Disorders Identification Test: Guidelines for Use in Primary Care. Available at: http://whqlibdoc.who.int/hq/2001/who_msd_msb_01.6a.pdf. Accessed June 16, 2011.

20. Rollman BL, Belnap BH, Mazumdar S, et al. A randomized trial to improve the quality of treatment for panic and generalized anxiety disorders in primary care. *Archives of General Psychiatry*. 2005;62(12):1332-41.

21. Kapczinski F, Lima MS, Souza JS, et al. Antidepressants for generalized anxiety disorder. *Cochrane Database Syst Rev*. 2003(2):CD003592.

22. Furukawa TA, Watanabe N, Churchill R. Combined psychotherapy plus antidepressants for panic disorder with or without agoraphobia. *Cochrane Database Syst Rev*. 2007(1):CD004364.

23. Haynes RB, Wilczynski NL. Optimal search strategies for retrieving scientifically strong studies of diagnosis from Medline: analytical survey. *BMJ*. 2004;328(7447):1040.

24. Wilczynski NL, Haynes RB. EMBASE search strategies for identifying methodologically sound diagnostic studies for use by clinicians and researchers. *BMC Med*. 2005;3:7.

25. Hsiao CJ, Cherry DK, Beatty PC, et al. National Ambulatory Medical Care Survey: 2007 summary. *Natl Health Stat Report*. 2010(27):1-32. Available at: http://www.cdc.gov/nchs/data/nhsr/nhsr027.pdf. Accessed August 8, 2011.

26. Bossuyt PM, Reitsma JB, Bruns DE, et al. The STARD statement for reporting studies of diagnostic accuracy: explanation and elaboration. *Ann Intern Med*. 2003;138(1):W1-12.

27. Whiting P, Rutjes AW, Reitsma JB, et al. The development of QUADAS: a tool for the quality assessment of studies of diagnostic accuracy included in systematic reviews. *BMC Med Res Methodol*. 2003;3:25.

28. Whiting PF, Weswood ME, Rutjes AW, et al. Evaluation of QUADAS, a tool for the quality assessment of diagnostic accuracy studies. *BMC Med Res Methodol*. 2006;6:9.

29. Higgins JP, Thompson SG, Deeks JJ, et al. Measuring inconsistency in meta-analyses. *BMJ*. 2003;327(7414):557-60.

30. Zamora J, Abraira V, Muriel A, et al. Meta-DiSc: a software for meta-analysis of test accuracy data. *BMC Med Res Methodol*. 2006;6:31.

31. Wallace BC, Schmid CH, Lau J, et al. Meta-Analyst: software for meta-analysis of binary, continuous and diagnostic data. *BMC Med Res Methodol*. 2009;9:80.

32.   Kincaid JP, Fishburne RP, Rogers RL, et al. *Derivation of New Readability Formulas (Automated Readability Index, Fog Count and Flesch Reading Ease Formula) for Navy Enlisted Personnel.* Naval Technical Training Command Millington Tenn Research Branch; 1975.

33.   Schunemann HJ, Oxman AD, Brozek J, et al. Grading quality of evidence and strength of recommendations for diagnostic tests and strategies. *BMJ*. 2008;336(7653):1106-10.

34.   Krasucki C, Ryan P, Ertan T, et al. The FEAR: A rapid screening instrument for generalized anxiety in elderly primary care attenders. *Int J Geriatr Psychiatry*. 1999;14(1):60-68.

35.   Spitzer RL, Kroenke K, Williams JB, et al. A brief measure for assessing generalized anxiety disorder: the GAD-7. *Arch Intern Med*. 2006;166(10):1092-7.

36.   Barsky AJ, Ahern DK, Delamater BA, et al. Differential diagnosis of palpitations. Preliminary development of a screening instrument. *Arch Fam Med*. 1997;6(3):241-5.

37.   Johnson MR, Hartzema AG, Mills TL, et al. Ethnic differences in the reliability and validity of a Panic Disorder Screen. *Ethn Health*. 2007;12(3):283-96.

38.   Spitzer RL, Williams JB, Kroenke K, et al. Utility of a new procedure for diagnosing mental disorders in primary care. The PRIME-MD 1000 study. *JAMA*. 1994;272(22):1749-56.

39.   Leon AC, Olfson M, Weissman MM, et al. Brief screens for mental disorders in primary care. *J Gen Intern Med*. 1996;11(7):426-30.

40.   Broadhead WE, Leon AC, Weissman MM, et al. Development and validation of the SDDS-PC screen for multiple mental disorders in primary care. *Arch Fam Med*. 1995;4(3):211-9.

41.   Beck AT, Steer RA, Ball R, et al. Use of the Beck Anxiety and Depression Inventories for primary care with medical outpatients. *Assessment*. 1997;4(3):211-219.

42.   Beck AT, Epstein N, Brown G, et al. An inventory for measuring clinical anxiety: psychometric properties. *J Consult Clin Psychol*. 1988;56(6):893-7.

43.   Wing JK. A technique for studying psychiatric morbidity in in-patient and out-patient series and in general population samples. *Psychol Med*. 1976;6(4):665-71.

44.   Reiss S, Peterson RA, Gursky DM, et al. Anxiety sensitivity, anxiety frequency and the prediction of fearfulness. *Behav Res Ther*. 1986;24(1):1-8.

45.   Apfeldorf WJ, Shear MK, Leon AC, et al. A brief screen for panic disorder. *Journal of Anxiety Disorders*;8(1):71-78.

46.   Mori DL, Lambert JF, Niles BL, et al. The BAI–PC as a Screen for Anxiety, Depression, and PTSD in Primary Care. *Journal of Clinical Psychology in Medical Settings*. 2003;10(3):187-192.

47.   Gunning R. *The technique of clear writing*. Rev. ed New York,: McGraw-Hill; 1968.

48.   Johnson MR, Hartzema AG, Mills TL, et al. Ethnic differences in the reliability and validity of a Panic Disorder Screen. *Ethn Health*. 2007;12(3):283-96.

49.   Kobak KA, Taylor LH, Dottl SL, et al. A computer-administered telephone interview to identify mental disorders. *JAMA*. 1997;278(11):905-10.

50.   Pinto-Meza A, Serrano-Blanco A, Penarrubia MT, et al. Assessing depression in primary care with the PHQ-9: can it be carried out over the telephone? *J Gen Intern Med*. 2005;20(8):738-42.

51.   Anonymous. Generalised anxiety disorder and panic disorder (with or without agoraphobia) in adults: management in primary, secondary and community care (partial update). National Clinical Guideline Number 113. National Collaborating Centre for Mental Health and the Royal College of General Practitioners. Commissioned by the National Institute for Health and Clinical Excellence. Available at: http://www.nice.org.uk/nicemedia/live/13314/52667/52667.pdf. Accessed June 13, 2011.

52.   Hunot V, Churchill R, Silva de Lima M, et al. Psychological therapies for generalised anxiety disorder. *Cochrane Database Syst Rev*. 2007(1):CD001848.

53.   Bakker A, van Balkom AJ, Spinhoven P. SSRIs vs. TCAs in the treatment of panic disorder: a meta-analysis. *Acta Psychiatr Scand*. 2002;106(3):163-7.

54.   Otto MW, Tuby KS, Gould RA, et al. An effect-size analysis of the relative efficacy and tolerability of serotonin selective reuptake inhibitors for panic disorder. *Am J Psychiatry*. 2001;158(12):1989-92.

55.   Clark DM, Salkovskis PM, Hackmann A, et al. Brief cognitive therapy for panic disorder: a randomized controlled trial. *J Consult Clin Psychol*. 1999;67(4):583-9.

56.   Carlbring P, Nilsson-Ihrfelt E, Waara J, et al. Treatment of panic disorder: live therapy vs. self-help via the Internet. *Behav Res Ther*. 2005;43(10):1321-33.

57.   American Psychiatric Association. DSM 5 Development. Available at: http://www.dsm5.org/ProposedRevision/Pages/proposedrevision.aspx?rid=167. Accessed June 17, 2011.

58.   Tatsioni A, Zarin DA, Aronson N, et al. Challenges in systematic reviews of diagnostic technologies. *Ann Intern Med*. 2005;142(12 Pt 2):1048-55.

59.   Pilkonis PA, Choi SW, Reise SP, et al. Item Banks for Measuring Emotional Distress From the Patient-Reported Outcomes Measurement Information System (PROMIS(R)): Depression, Anxiety, and Anger. *Assessment*. 2011.

60.   Mohlman J, Bryant C, Lenze EJ, et al. Improving recognition of late life anxiety disorders in Diagnostic and Statistical Manual of Mental Disorders, Fifth Edition: observations and recommendations of the Advisory Committee to the Lifespan Disorders Work Group. *Int J Geriatr Psychiatry*. 2011.

APPENDIX A. SEARCH STRATEGY

Step	Category	Terms	Result[a]
1	**Disorders**	(generalized AND anxiety AND disorder[tiab]) OR panic disorder[tiab] OR "generalized anxiety disorder" OR panic disorder[mesh] OR panic[title/abstract]	12293
2	**Measurement instruments**		
	GAD or PD	"gad7"[tiab] OR "generalized anxiety disorder 7"[tiab] OR "gad-7"[tiab] OR "beck anxiety"[tiab] OR "geriatric anxiety inventory"[tiab] OR "short anxiety screening test"[tiab] OR "hospital anxiety and depression scale"[tiab] OR PHQ[tiab] OR "patient health questionnaire"[tiab] OR "zung anxiety scale"[tiab] OR "penn state worry questionnaire"[tiab] OR "multicenter collaborative panic disorder severity scale"	3801
	Broad terms for instruments	**OR** "Psychiatric Status Rating Scales"[Mesh] OR questionnaires[MeSH Terms] OR questionnaires[tiab] OR questionnaire[tiab] OR tools[tiab] OR tool[tiab] OR scale[tiab] OR scales[tiab] OR inventory[tiab] OR screening[tiab]	1,094,242
3	**Instrument characteristics**	medical history taking[mh] OR reproducibility of results[mh] OR observer variation[mh] OR sensitivity[tiab] OR specificity[tiab] OR "sensitivity and specificity"[mh] OR likelihood [tiab] OR accura*[tiab]	1,249,615
4	**Combine results and apply limits**	#1 AND #2 AND #3 English and Human and Adult	850

[a]Numbers reflect the result of the PubMed search only.

APPENDIX B. STUDY SELECTION FORM

INCLUSION CRITERIA:

- Sample population is adults age ≥18 years presenting with a somatic symptom or presenting to a medical clinic for a scheduled appointment.

- Setting is primary care (general internal medicine, family medicine, geriatrics) or general medical (emergency department, women's health clinic).

- Intervention is a self-report instrument (index test) designed to screen for or facilitate diagnosis of GAD, PD, or anxiety disorders. The instrument must be feasible in a clinical setting without requiring special equipment and may be performed by a nonexpert.

- Reference standard diagnosis of GAD or PD is made using acceptable criteria (e.g., DSM-III or later, ICD-9 or later) and administered by a trained clinician.

- Study reports a measure of reliability or sensitivity/specificity or the data to calculate at least one of these performance characteristics.

- Study design is prospective comparison of an anxiety questionnaire to a reference standard; reference standard must be applied to all subjects or to a randomly selected subsample that allows correction for verification bias.

- Study must be published in a peer-reviewed publication.

EXCLUSION CRITERIA:

- Study is a non-English language publication. English language articles that address Spanish version of instruments will be included.

- Study is conducted outside of North America, Western Europe, New Zealand or Australia.

- Study populations are patients with current mental illness (e.g., substance abuse disorder), and screening is for comorbid anxiety disorder.

- Anxiety measure and reference standard are performed by the same individual.

Performance Characteristics of Self-report Instruments for Diagnosing Generalized Anxiety and Panic Disorders in Primary Care

Evidence-based Synthesis Program

APPENDIX C. EXCLUDED STUDIES

All studies listed below were reviewed in their full-text version and excluded for the reason indicated. An alphabetical reference list follows the table.

Reference	Population not of interest	Setting not PC, clinic, or ER	No self-reported index test at screening	Reference standard not acceptable	No instrument characteristics data	Design not prospective	Reference standard not applied correctly	Publication not English	Screening tool not English/Spanish
Andersson, 2004 (422)		X							
Andjreu, 2008 (1551)	X								
Andreescu, 2008 (124)						X			
Apfeldorf, 1994 (1690)	X								
Argyropoulos, 2007 (247)		X							
Austin, 2006 (321)		X							
Baughman, 1994 (2675)			X						
Beck, 1996 (801)		X							
Behar, 2003 (505)		X							
Berrocal, 2006 (316)		X							
Berrocal, 2006 (362)		X							
Bieling, 1998 (721)		X							
Bobes, 2006 (315)								X	
Bucholz, 1991 (2532)	X								
Bystritsky, 1996 (810)		X							
Clum, 1990 (3010)	X								
Connor, 2001 (2399)	X								
Dammen, 1999 (674)								X	
Eack, 2006 (1478)		X							
Eack, 2008 (149)		X							
Epstein, 2001 (2417)		X							
Farvolden, 2003 (486)		X							
Fleet, 1997 (759)								X	
Gladstone, 2005 (345)	X								
Gloster, 2008 (174)	X								
Jackson, 2007 (243)					X				
Kobak, 1997 (751)	X								
Kuijpers, 2003 (497)							X		
Lowe, 2003 (477)									X
Lykouras, 1996 (2256)		X							

Performance Characteristics of Self-report Instruments for Diagnosing Generalized Anxiety and Panic Disorders in Primary Care

Reference	Population not of interest	Setting not PC, clinic, or ER	No self-reported index test at screening	Reference standard not acceptable	No instrument characteristics data	Design not prospective	Reference standard not applied correctly	Publication not English	Screening tool not English/ Spanish
McQuaid, 2000 (633)							X		
Means–Christensen 2005 (343)				X					
Means–Christensen, 2006 (319)	X								
Meyer, 1990 (946)		X							
Mori, 2003 (3846)				X					
Morlock, 2008 (190)	X								
Mowry, 1990 (2735)		X							
Mussell, 2008 (150)	X	X							
Newman, 2006 (310)	X								
Novy, 2001 (587)	X								
Olsson, 2005 (1625)				X					
Parker, 1997 (747)	X								
Parkerson, 1997 (767)				X					
Robinson, 2010 (1021)		X							
Rollman, 2005 (371)							X		
Sandin, 1996 (800)	X								
Senior, 2007 (3868)	X								
Stein, 1999 (2268)							X		
Svanborg, 1994 (872)	X								
Vujanovic, 2007 (227)				X					
Webb, 2008 (114)	X								
Weissman, 1998 (735)			X						
Wetherell, 2007 (271)		X							
Yingling, 1993 (886)					X				

LIST OF EXCLUDED STUDIES

Andersson G, Carlbring P, Kaldo V, et al. Screening of psychiatric disorders via the Internet. A pilot study with tinnitus patients. *Nord J Psychiatry*. 2004;58(4):287-91.

Andjreu Y, Galdón MJ, Dura E, et al. Psychometric properties of the Brief Symptoms Inventory-18 (BSI-18) in a Spanish sample of outpatients with psychiatric disorders. *Psicothema*. 2008;20(4):844-850.

Andreescu C, Belnap BH, Rollman BL, et al. Generalized anxiety disorder severity scale validation in older adults. *Am J Geriatr Psychiatry*. 2008;16(10):813-8.

Apfeldorf WJ, Shear MK, Leon AC, et al. A brief screen for panic disorder. *Journal of Anxiety Disorders*. 1994;8(1):71-78.

Argyropoulos SV, Ploubidis GB, Wright TS, et al. Development and validation of the Generalized Anxiety Disorder Inventory (GADI). *J Psychopharmacol*. 2007;21(2):145-52.

Austin DW, Richards JC, Klein B. Modification of the Body Sensations Interpretation Questionnaire (BSIQ-M): validity and reliability. *Journal of Anxiety Disorders*. 2006;20(2):237-51.

Baughman OL. Rapid diagnosis and treatment of anxiety and depression in primary care: The somatizing patient. *The Journal of Family Practice*. 1994;39(4):373-378.

Beck JG, Stanley MA, Zebb BJ. Characteristics of generalized anxiety disorder in older adults: a descriptive study. *Behav Res Ther*. 1996;34(3):225-34.

Behar E, Alcaine O, Zuellig AR, et al. Screening for generalized anxiety disorder using the Penn State Worry Questionnaire: a receiver operating characteristic analysis. *J Behav Ther Exp Psychiatry*. 2003;34(1):25-43.

Berrocal C, Ruiz Moreno M, Merchan P, et al. The Mood Spectrum Self-Report: validation and adaptation into Spanish. *Depress Anxiety*. 2006;23(4):220-35.

Berrocal C, Ruiz Moreno MA, Gil Villa M, et al. Multidimensional assessment of the Panic-Agoraphobic Spectrum: reliability and validity of the Spanish version of the PAS-SR. *Journal of Anxiety Disorders*. 2006;20(5):562-79.

Bieling PJ, Antony MM, Swinson RP. The State-Trait Anxiety Inventory, Trait version: structure and content re-examined. *Behav Res Ther*. 1998;36(7-8):777-88.

Bobes J, Garcia-Calvo C, Prieto R, et al. Psychometric properties of the Spanish version of the screening scale for DSM-IV Generalized Anxiety Disorder of Carroll and Davidson. *Actas Esp Psiquiatr*. 2006;34(2):83-93.

Bucholz KK, Robins LN, Shayka JJ, et al. Performance of two forms of a computer psychiatric screening interview: Version I of the DISSI. *J Psychiatr Res*. 1991;25(3):117-129.

Bystritsky A, Waikar SV, Vapnik T. Four-dimensional Anxiety and Depression Scale: a preliminary psychometric report. *Anxiety*. 1996;2(1):47-50.

Clum GA, Broyles S, Borden J, et al. Validity and reliability of the panic attack symptoms and cognitions questionnaires. *Journal of Psychopathology and Behavioral Assessment*. 1990;12(3):233-245.

Connor KM, Kobak KA, Churchill LE, et al. Mini-SPIN: A brief screening assessment for generalized social anxiety disorder. *Depress Anxiety*. 2001;14(2):137-140.

Dammen T, Ekeberg O, Arnesen H, et al. The detection of panic disorder in chest pain patients. *Gen Hosp Psychiatry*. 1999;21(5):323-32.

Eack SM, Greeno CG, Lee B-J. Limitations of the Patient Health Questionnaire in Identifying Anxiety and Depression in Community Mental Health: Many Cases are Undetected. *Research on Social Work Practice*. 2006;16(6):625-631.

Eack SM, Singer JB, Greeno CG. Screening for anxiety and depression in community mental health: the beck anxiety and depression inventories. *Community Ment Health J.* 2008;44(6):465-74.

Epstein JF, Barker PR, Kroutil LA. Mode effects in self-reported mental health data. *Public Opin Q.* 2001;65(4):529-549.

Farvolden P, McBride C, Bagby RM, et al. A Web-based screening instrument for depression and anxiety disorders in primary care. *J Med Internet Res.* 2003;5(3):e23.

Fleet RP, Dupuis G, Marchand A, et al. Detecting panic disorder in emergency department chest pain patients: a validated model to improve recognition. *Ann Behav Med.* 1997;19(2):124-31.

Gladstone GL, Parker GB, Mitchell PB, et al. A Brief Measure of Worry Severity (BMWS): personality and clinical correlates of severe worriers. *Journal of Anxiety Disorders.* 2005;19(8):877-92.

Gloster AT, Rhoades HM, Novy D, et al. Psychometric properties of the Depression Anxiety and Stress Scale-21 in older primary care patients. *J Affect Disord.* 2008;110(3):248-59.

Jackson JL, Passamonti M, Kroenke K. Outcome and impact of mental disorders in primary care at 5 years. *Psychosom Med.* 2007;69(3):270-6.

Kobak KA, Taylor LH, Dottl SL, et al. Computerized screening for psychiatric disorders in an outpatient community mental health clinic. *Psychiatr Serv.* 1997;48(8):1048-57.

Kuijpers PM, Denollet J, Lousberg R, et al. Validity of the hospital anxiety and depression scale for use with patients with noncardiac chest pain. *Psychosomatics.* 2003;44(4):329-35.

Lowe B, Grafe K, Zipfel S, et al. Detecting panic disorder in medical and psychosomatic outpatients: comparative validation of the Hospital Anxiety and Depression Scale, the Patient Health Questionnaire, a screening question, and physicians' diagnosis. *J Psychosom Res.* 2003;55(6):515-9.

Lykouras L, Adrachta D, Kalfakis N, et al. GHQ-28 as an aid to detect mental disorders in neurological inpatients. *Acta Psychiatr Scand.* 1996;93(3):212-216.

McQuaid JR, Stein MB, McCahill M, et al. Use of brief psychiatric screening measures in a primary care sample. *Depress Anxiety.* 2000;12(1):21-9.

Means-Christensen AJ, Arnau RC, Tonidandel AM, et al. An efficient method of identifying major depression and panic disorder in primary care. *J Behav Med.* 2005;28(6):565-72.

Means-Christensen AJ, Sherbourne CD, Roy-Byrne PP, et al. Using five questions to screen for five common mental disorders in primary care: diagnostic accuracy of the Anxiety and Depression Detector. *Gen Hosp Psychiatry.* 2006;28(2):108-18.

Meyer TJ, Miller ML, Metzger RL, et al. Development and validation of the Penn State Worry Questionnaire. *Behav Res Ther.* 1990;28(6):487-95.

Mori DL, Lambert JF, Niles BL, et al. The BAI–PC as a Screen for Anxiety, Depression, and PTSD in Primary Care. *Journal of Clinical Psychology in Medical Settings.* 2003;10(3):187-192.

Morlock RJ, Williams VS, Cappelleri JC, et al. Development and evaluation of the Daily Assessment of Symptoms - Anxiety (DAS-A) scale to evaluate onset of symptom relief in patients with generalized anxiety disorder. *J Psychiatr Res.* 2008;42(12):1024-36.

Mowry BJ, Burvill PW. Screening the elderly in the community for psychiatric disorder. *Aust N Z J Psychiatry.* 1990;24(2):203-206.

Mussell M, Kroenke K, Spitzer RL, et al. Gastrointestinal symptoms in primary care: prevalence and association with depression and anxiety. *J Psychosom Res.* 2008;64(6):605-12.

Newman MG, Holmes M, Zuellig AR, et al. The reliability and validity of the panic disorder self-report: a new diagnostic screening measure of panic disorder. *Psychol Assess.* 2006;18(1):49-61.

Novy DM, Stanley MA, Averill P, et al. Psychometric comparability of English- and Spanish-language measures of anxiety and related affective symptoms. *Psychol Assess.* 2001;13(3):347-55.

Olssøn I, Mykletun A, Dahl AA. The hospital anxiety and depression rating scale: A cross-sectional study of psychometrics and case finding abilities in general practice. *BMC Psychiatry.* 2005;5.

Parker G, Roussos J, Hadzi-Pavlovic D, et al. The development of a refined measure of dysfunctional parenting and assessment of its relevance in patients with affective disorders. *Psychol Med.* 1997;27(5):1193-203.

Parkerson GR, Jr., Broadhead WE. Screening for anxiety and depression in primary care with the Duke Anxiety-Depression Scale. *Fam Med.* 1997;29(3):177-81.

Robinson CM, Klenck SC, Norton PJ. Psychometric properties of the Generalized Anxiety Disorder Questionnaire for DSM-IV among four racial groups. *Cognitive Behaviour Therapy.* 2010;39(4):251-261.

Rollman BL, Belnap BH, Mazumdar S, et al. Symptomatic severity of PRIME-MD diagnosed episodes of panic and generalized anxiety disorder in primary care. *J Gen Intern Med.* 2005;20(7):623-8.

Senior, A.C, Kunik, M.E, Rhoades, H.M, et al. Utility of telephone assessments in an older adult population. *Psychol Aging.* 2007:22(2): p. 392-7.

Sandin B, Chorot P, McNally RJ. Validation of the Spanish version of the Anxiety Sensitivity Index in a clinical sample. *Behav Res Ther.* 1996;34(3):283-90.

Stein MB, Jang KL, Livesley WJ. Heritability of anxiety sensitivity: A twin study. *The American Journal of Psychiatry.* 1999;156(2):246-251.

Svanborg P, Asberg M. A new self-rating scale for depression and anxiety states based on the Comprehensive Psychopathological Rating Scale. *Acta Psychiatr Scand.* 1994;89(1):21-8.

Vujanovic AA, Arrindell WA, Bernstein A, et al. Sixteen-item Anxiety Sensitivity Index: confirmatory factor analytic evidence, internal consistency, and construct validity in a young adult sample from the Netherlands. *Assessment.* 2007;14(2):129-43.

Webb SA, Diefenbach G, Wagener P, et al. Comparison of self-report measures for identifying late-life generalized anxiety in primary care. *J Geriatr Psychiatry Neurol.* 2008;21(4):223-31.

Weissman MM, Broadhead WE, Olfson M, et al. A diagnostic aid for detecting (DSM-IV) mental disorders in primary care. *Gen Hosp Psychiatry.* 1998;20(1):1-11.

Wetherell JL, Birchler GD, Ramsdell J, et al. Screening for generalized anxiety disorder in geriatric primary care patients. *Int J Geriatr Psychiatry.* 2007;22(2):115-23.

Yingling KW, Wulsin LR, Arnold LM, et al. Estimated prevalences of panic disorder and depression among consecutive patients seen in an emergency department with acute chest pain. *J Gen Intern Med.* 1993;8(5):231-5.

APPENDIX D. DATA EXTRACTION FORM

Data abstraction for anxiety screening in primary care

Reviewer initials   Endnote ref #:
First Author: Year Published: Country:
Primary study: 1) Yes   2)No.   Linked study: 1) Yes   2) No

I) Study setting

1)Outpatient primary care clinic   2) Specialty clinic (specify):

3)ER   4)OB/GYN or women's health

Comments:

II) Patient presentation: Did the patients present with a physical symptoms

1)Chest pain   2)Unselected   3)Other Symptom: 4)NR-99

III) Type of setting   NR -99

1) Academic   2) Community   3) Mixed
4) Other (specify):

Comments:

IV) VA clinics   NR -99   1) Only VA   2) Mixed   3) No VA

V) Selection of population for screening   NR -99

1) Random   2)Consecutive   3)Convenience
4) Other (specify)

Comments:

VI) Selection of population for criterion standard   NR -99

1) Random   2)Consecutive   3)Convenience
4) Other (specify)

Comments:

VII) Description of study population   NR -99

Comments:

Potentially eligible: N=

Met eligibility criteria: N=

Screened: N=

Completed criterion standard:

VIII) Age   NR-99   (Age is for results not for selection)

Mean age (SD)

Age range:

Comments:

IX) Gender   NR-99

Male (n)=

Female (n)=

Comments:

X) Ethnicity   NR-99

1) Caucasian N=   2) Black N=

3) Hispanic N =   4) Asian N=

5) Other N=

Comments:

XI) Education   NR-99

Mean years completed (±SD):

Other measures:

Comments:

XII) Name of the screening instrument (specify version and number when applicable: eg GAD-7 OR GAD-2)

XIII) Methods of administration of screening test   NR-99

1) Self-administered   2) Interviewer administered   3) Via telephone

4) Computer assisted   5) Other (specify):

XIV) What was the criterion standard   NR-99

1) DSM IV   2) DSM IIIR   3) DSM III   4) ICD 9/10

5) Research diagnostic criteria (RDC)   6) Other (specify)

XV) Method used to determining standard   NR-99

1) SCID   2)DIS   3)CIDI   4)DSM3/4   5)ADIS   6) Other (specify):

XVI) Medical comorbidity: specific diseases or average measures   1) Yes   NR-99

List top 3 or measures:

XVII) Psychiatric comorbidity   1) Yes   NR-99

	Excluded	(1)	<10%	(2)	10-25%	(3)	>25%	(4)	NR (-99)
Depression									
PTSD									
Substance abuse									
Social anxiety									
GAD									
PD									
Other ( )									
Other ( )									

XVIII) Other measures:

Responsiveness: NR-99

Test retest reliability: NR-99

RESULTS

Total sample/ Subgroup . If subgroup, specify:

Test used to detect   1)GAD   2)PD   3) Both   Results for multiple cutoffs given: 1) Yes   2)No

Cutoff picked a priori?   1)Yes   2) No   Same as traditional cutoff: 1) Yes   2) No

Gold standard ↓

	pos	neg	
pos co= ( )			
neg co= ( )			

Other measures, eg sensitivity, PPV, LR: (give 95% CI or NR-99)

Statistic:	Data	95% CI

Data validated?   1) Yes   2) No   Data adjusted for sampling: 1) Yes   2) No

Total sample/ Subgroup . If subgroup, specify:

2) Test used to detect   1)GAD   2)PD   3) Both   Results for multiple cutoffs given: 1) Yes   2)No

Cutoff picked a priori?   1)Yes   2) No   Same as traditional cutoff: 1) Yes   2) No

Gold standard ↓

	pos	neg	
pos co= ( )			
neg co= ( )			

Other Measures., eg sensitivity, PPV, LR: (give 95% CI or NR-99)

Statistic:	Data	95% CI

Data validated?   1) Yes   2) No   Data adjusted for sampling: 1) Yes   2) No

43

Total sample/ Subgroup . If subgroup, specify:

Test used to detect 1)GAD 2)PD 3) Both   Results for multiple cutoffs given: 1) Yes 2)No

Cutoff picked a priori? 1)Yes 2) No   Same as traditional cutoff: 1) Yes 2) No

Gold standard ↓

	pos	neg	
pos co= ( )			
neg co= ( )			

Other Measures., eg sensitivity, PPV, LR: (give 95% CI or NR-99)

Statistic:	Data	95% CI

Data validated? 1) Yes 2) No

Total sample/ Subgroup . If subgroup, specify:

Test used to detect 1)GAD 2)PD 3) Both   Results for multiple cutoffs given: 1) Yes 2)No

Cutoff picked a priori? 1)Yes 2) No   Same as traditional cutoff: 1) Yes 2) No

Gold standard ↓

	pos	neg	
pos co= ( )			
neg co= ( )			

Other Measures., eg sensitivity, PPV, LR: (give 95% CI or NR-99)

Statistic:	Data	95% CI

Data validated? 1) Yes 2) No

Inclusion and Exclusion Criteria:

APPENDIX E. CRITERIA USED IN QUALITY ASSESSMENT

QUADAS tool* with modified item 12.

Item	Yes	No	Unclear
1. Was the spectrum of patients representative of the patients who will receive the test in practice?	( )	( )	( )
2. Were selection criteria clearly described?	( )	( )	( )
3. Is the reference standard likely to correctly classify the target condition?	( )	( )	( )
4. Is the time period between reference standard and index test short enough to be reasonably sure that the target condition did not change between the two tests? (Yes if one month or less)	( )	( )	( )
5. Did the whole sample or a random selection of the sample, receive verification using a reference standard of diagnosis?	( )	( )	( )
6. Did patients receive the same reference standard regardless of the index test result?	( )	( )	( )
7. Was the reference standard independent of the index test (i.e. the index test did not form part of the reference standard)?	( )	( )	( )
8. Was the execution of the index test described in sufficient detail to permit replication of the test?	( )	( )	( )
9. Was the execution of the reference standard described in sufficient detail to permit its replication?	( )	( )	( )
10. Were the index test results interpreted without knowledge of the results of the reference standard?	( )	( )	( )
11. Were the reference standard results interpreted without knowledge of the results of the index test?	( )	( )	( )
12. Was the cut off point for the test chosen a priori?	( )	( )	( )
13. Were uninterpretable/intermediate test results including missing data reported?	( )	( )	( )
14. Were withdrawals from the study explained?	( )	( )	( )

Whiting PF, Weswood ME, Rutjes AW, Reitsma JB, Bossuyt PN, Kleijnen J. Evaluation of QUADAS, a tool for the quality assessment of diagnostic accuracy studies. *BMC Med Res Methodol.* 2006;6:9.

Performance Characteristics of Self-report Instruments for Diagnosing
Generalized Anxiety and Panic Disorders in Primary Care

Evidence-based Synthesis Program

APPENDIX F. PEER REVIEW COMMENTS/AUTHOR RESPONSES

Reviewer	Comment	Response
Question 1: Are the objectives, scope, and methods for this review clearly described?		
1	Yes	Thank you.
2	Yes- The topic is important and is clearly justified in the introduction. The scope is clearly described. I was a bit disappointed that the scope did not include assessment of anxiety in the context of depression, given the high comorbidity. The authors did an exceptional job of writing methods that were easy for this reader to follow.	Thank you. Including studies that assess the performance of anxiety measures in patients with concurrent depression is an excellent idea. We did not encounter any such studies conducted in primary care settings. A future report could include a broader range of settings that might include this population.
3	Yes - Methodology is clearly described and appropriate to the question asked.	Thank you.
4	Yes- From these, we identified no recent systematic reviews and 12 observational reports on 9 unique studies that addressed one of the key questions. This sentence isn't clear to me; is it: 1) No systematic reviews; 2) 12 observational reports; 3) 9 unique studies?	We have changed this sentence to read "12 articles from 9 unique studies…" to clarify that there were nine studies, some of which had more than one resulting publication.
5	Yes	Thank you.
6	Yes- The objectives are clear-cut, and the review clarifies the potential and considerable limitations of prior research on screening tools for GAD and panic disorder. This report is timely and of great importance. The authors correctly point out that GAD and panic disorder are quite common mental illnesses in the VA population, with considerable impairment in quality of life and physical and cognitive health, and that treatments – SSRIs, other antidepressants, and CBT (all quite implementable within the VA health care system) – are effective for these common and typically undetected conditions. In my own opinion, the lack of detection of these anxiety disorders within the health care system is one of the "low-hanging fruit" in which to improve mental health treatment.	Thank you.
7	No- See my comment below re: Page 8, Table 1 inclusion and exclusion criteria and how they relate to KQ1.	Acknowledged
Question 2: Is there any indication of bias in our synthesis of the evidence?		
1	No	Acknowledged
2	No- There is no evidence of bias in the data synthesis.	Thank you.

46

Performance Characteristics of Self-report Instruments for Diagnosing Generalized Anxiety and Panic Disorders in Primary Care

Evidence-based Synthesis Program

Reviewer	Comment	Response
3	No- Authors' disclosures indicate no overt bias. In selecting articles, they did exclude non-English-language measures and articles, possibly excluding high-quality studies, though it is true the excluded studies would likely have been less applicable to the VHA population. As the authors point out, there is some possibility of publication bias, as there is no trials register for diagnostic studies; inasmuch as possible, the search strategy was thorough and comprehensive.	Unfortunately, our resource limitations do not permit bilingual staff or translation services. Since foreign language publications often deal with foreign language questionnaires and this report was written to serve a Veteran population in the United States, we do not think we have missed many pertinent articles. We acknowledge the language limitation in the discussion.
4	No	Acknowledged
5	No	Acknowledged
6	Yes -None	Thank you.
7	No	Acknowledged
Question 3: Are there any studies of interest to the VA that we have overlooked?		
1	No	Acknowledged
2	No, I performed a separate search, particularly looking for anxiety assessment in the elderly, and I could find no studies that were not already included.	Thank you for checking our work! We are glad we did not miss key studies.
3	Yes- Non-English language articles (these studies were excluded).	Unfortunately, our resource limitations do not permit bilingual staff or translation services. Since foreign language publications often deal with foreign language questionnaires and this report was written to serve a Veteran population in the United States, we do not think we have missed many pertinent articles. We acknowledge the language limitation in the discussion.
4	No	Acknowledged
5	No- Search strategy documented in report appears thorough.	Thank you.
6	Yes. The DSM-V workgroup on late-life anxiety disorders has recently published a review of the difficulties of detecting anxiety disorders in older adults. Within this review are some potentially helpful recommendations for improving the characteristics of screening and diagnostic measures for this difficult to assess population (due to insight and memory problems). The citation is Mohlman et al, International Journal of Geriatric Psychiatry. If it is not yet available, you could get it directly from the 1st author, Jan Mohlman, Ph.D., jmohlman@rci.rutgers. edu.	Thank you for this suggestion. We have cited this article in our discussion.
7	No	Acknowledged

Performance Characteristics of Self-report Instruments for Diagnosing
Generalized Anxiety and Panic Disorders in Primary Care

Evidence-based Synthesis Program

Reviewer	Comment	Response
Question 4: Are there any clinical performance measures, programs, quality improvement measures, patient care services, or conferences that will be directly affected by this report? If so, please provide detail.		
1	PACT and associated programs (e.g., primary care-mental health integration) are directly relevant to these results. Casefinding, identification of comorbid anxiety disorders, and tracking treatment progress (i.e., measurement-based care) are important activities for these programs.	We have revised the discussion to identify specific programs (e.g. PACT, primary care-mental health integration) that may want to the recommended instruments. As none of the instruments have been tested for response to change, we think it is too early to implement them for monitoring treatment response.
2	Given the review did not find one measure superior to others, it is not clear that this report will effect an immediate change in these areas. The report does highlight the need for future research on outcomes of anxiety screening.	Based on feasibility and performance characteristics, we identified and recommended the most promising instruments. We have noted the need for further research on the effects of routine screening for anxiety disorders.
3	No comment	Acknowledged
4	Not aware of any	Acknowledged
5	No. Report does not appear to recommend any additions to VA services at this time. However, report makes no practical recommendations so this question is hard to answer.	We have revised the report to make more explicit recommendations, including a summary table of recommendations.
6	I am insufficiently familiar with the VA programs to fully answer this, but it appears that the key conclusion from this report is that there is insufficient evidence regarding the value of existing screening methods for these disorders in VA settings (especially primary care). The logical conclusion would be to recommend to the VA HSR&D that a funding opportunity be made to create and test screening methods.	Thank you for your comment. We are assured that the report will be widely disseminated within the VA system. We have also included a specific recommendation for VA R&D to consider supporting studies on anxiety measures and anxiety screening.
7	No comment	Acknowledged
Question 5: Please provide any recommendations on how this report can be revised to more directly address or assist implementation needs.		
1	While the immediate and explicit aims of the report are specifically framed and very nicely accomplished, addition or further discussion of three issues could be made in several places (namely, framing the questions up front, recommending future research directions, and suggesting implementation needs) to further enhance the utility of this report or inform future work. Specifically, these three issues are: 1) the known or unknown science and the advisability on a practical level of using measures for following treatment progress in addition to casefinding; 2) the role of phone administration in future research; and 3) advice for implementation or research on the best clinical or population contexts for using these instruments for efficient and effective casefinding in general medical settings.	1) This is a very good point and idea. Our review did not specifically address the advisability of measurement-based care but we cite two anxiety care management studies that used this approach with positive results. 2) This is also a very good point, and we have amended the report to address it to a limited degree in the Recommendation for Future Research section as well as in the Summary of Recommendations. 3) We revised the discussion to comment on current recommended uses and the research on the performance of anxiety measures in specific populations.

**Performance Characteristics of Self-report Instruments for Diagnosing
Generalized Anxiety and Panic Disorders in Primary Care**

Evidence-based Synthesis Program

Reviewer	Comment	Response
2	As indicated above, the report might include some comment about screening for anxiety among depressives and comorbidity of these illnesses.	We discussed the potential for change in performance in individuals with depressive or medical illness. In addition, we commented on applicability to specific VA programs.
3	Given the important contribution of untreated mental illness to overall healthcare utilization and cost, reasonably effective and feasible diagnostic screening tools for patient self-administration in the medical setting could have an impact on overall health as well as healthcare expenditures. Use of screening tools for GAD and PD in primary care clinics may be an important first step; an algorithm for "what to do if the patient screens positive" might be helpful in encouraging implementation of a screening program.	We agree that such an algorithm would be highly useful if the policy implementation experts at the VA decide to start routine screening for anxiety disorders in primary care venues.
4	The report states: Patients referred to the integrated-care programs are also screened for comorbid conditions, including anxiety disorders. I'm not aware of screening for comorbid conditions including anxiety disorders in integrated care programs. If this were being done, it seems like we might have internal data to draw on or would have some information on what screening tools are being used.	The original call for proposals to establish mental health–primary care programs specified routine screening for anxiety disorders. However, these data are not being collected routinely at a national level. We will promote our report to the MH-PC program.
5	The methodology is sound and the evidence appears clear. The conclusions are theoretical and do not appear to provide any practical recommendations (e.g., that none of the measures examined should be implemented, that VA should devote funds to developing and researching new screening instruments, etc.). Also, it is unclear whether the overall VA policy will be to manage GAD and PD in primary care (hence necessitating a diagnostic instrument) or refer positive screens to Mental Health for more accurate diagnosis (which would necessitate only a brief screen, similar to the brief screenings VA uses now in primary care).	Thank you. We revised the report to offer more practical recommendations, including the need for research to inform the effects of screening in primary care. Making recommendations for VA policy—such as care for patients in primary care versus mental health settings—is beyond the scope of the report.

Performance Characteristics of Self-report Instruments for Diagnosing
Generalized Anxiety and Panic Disorders in Primary Care

Evidence-based Synthesis Program

Reviewer	Comment	Response
6	I have several comments. My apologies if some of these go beyond the stated purpose of the expert review:	
	It is likely that a screening instrument will need to do more than simply detect anxiety. It will need to diagnose and track the severity of these disorders, as providers in the VA system (other than psychologists) will not have the time, ability, or inclination to do these.	We agree that tracking responsiveness to change is an important attribute of a good screening instrument. However, the instruments included in the review have not been evaluated for sensitivity to change. Therefore, we included this as a recommendation for future research and have highlighted it again in the Summary of Recommendations section.
	My understanding is that the VA health care system has a lot of older adults. A particular focus is needed on whether the screening instruments would have adequate ability to detect anxiety disorders in this age group. Older adults are notoriously difficult to screen for and diagnose anxiety disorders, given memory and insight issues, among others.	The reviewer is correct in that the VA does have a lot of older adults in whom detection of anxiety disorders is challenging. We have amended the Recommendations for Future Research section of the report to highlight this point. We agree that changes in the diagnostic criteria can affect the performance of an instrument that has been validated using a different version of the DSM. This has been addressed Summary and Discussion section.
	Another comment is that the report does not seem to be taking the changes in these disorders with DSM-V into account. For example, will the GAD-7 still be relevant once GAD is revised into a disorder that more reflects the core concept of worry (and less the associated symptoms)?	The potential changes in the diagnosis of anxiety disorders resulting from the current discussions about diagnostic boundaries are pertinent. We have addressed the specificity of scales under development in the Recommendations for Future Research section.
	Along this same line, there is increasingly a move to question the diagnostic boundaries of these disorders and instead focus on (in the case of anxiety disorders) core dimensions of pathological anxiety such as distress and avoidance. As a concrete example of this issue, wouldn't the VA be better off with an instrument that detected not only GAD but also "anxiety disorder NOS" in the context of substance abuse?	We have added a brief comment on the issue of developing and evaluating scales that detect general anxiety versus those that assess for specific disorders. There are tradeoffs for each decision.
	Finally, might the reviewers want to consider the PROMIS anxiety item banks in their review? To my knowledge, these have not been used in exactly the way the reviewers are examining, but they have been the most extensively psychometrically tested items for measuring anxiety symptoms. I've reviewed them in the past, and many of the items appear quite good – very effective at assessing both the presence and severity of pathological anxiety	Thank you for this suggestion. We contacted one of the investigators regarding the PROMIS scales and also reviewed their Web site. We also conducted a literature search for the PROMIS anxiety scale. It appears that the scale has not yet been validated in a primary care sample and, therefore, could not be included in this report.

Performance Characteristics of Self-report Instruments for Diagnosing Generalized Anxiety and Panic Disorders in Primary Care

Reviewer	Comment	Response
7	Discussion/conclusion sections: Include more of a discussion of implementation within VA settings. You provide a brief discussion of parallels with the PHQ-9 for depression, and expanding this discussion related to how the recommended screening tools could be implemented within VA settings could be helpful for policy makers and providers who will make use of the findings.	We have added our recommendations for current implementation, limited to case-finding and a recommendation for research to address systematic screening.
	Are there any recommendations for universal screening?	USPTF does not have a current recommendation on routine anxiety screening, and we have specifically noted the lack of a recommendation. We did not conduct a systematic review of the effect of anxiety screening; however, this is an important question for future research.
	Should certain tools be included in CPRS and administered to certain populations at certain intervals?	This is a good suggestion, and we have recommended that the most promising tools be added to the MH assistant.
Question 6: Please provide us with contact details of any additional individuals/stakeholders who should be made aware of this report.		
1	Andy Pomerantz	Thank you, we will make sure Dr. Pomerantz is aware of our report.
2	It may help to send this to Dr. Eric Lenze at Washington University, who is an expert on anxiety in the elderly. His email is lenzee@wustl.edu	Thank you. The report will be disseminated broadly.
3	As with all integrative (medical / mental health) work, this is important information for anyone involved in healthcare policy and reform.	Thank you.
4	No comment	Acknowledged
5	None that I can think of.	Acknowledged
6	The individuals cited above would be a good start.	Acknowledged
7	Use of the indicated screening tools should be implemented. This could be done at the national level through central office, or at the VISN or Chief of mental health level. The office(s) responsible for implementation should be made aware of this report.	Acknowledged. We are assured that the report will be widely circulated inside the VA system.
Question 7: Please write additional suggestions or comments below. If applicable, please indicate the page and line numbers from the draft report.		
1	No Comment	Acknowledged
2	A very well written report	Thank you.
3	No Comment	Acknowledged
4	No Comment	Acknowledged

Performance Characteristics of Self-report Instruments for Diagnosing
Generalized Anxiety and Panic Disorders in Primary Care

Evidence-based Synthesis Program

Reviewer	Comment	Response
5	As noted in comments from item 5 above, some consideration should be given to the context in which this literature examination is taking place (i.e., VA setting versus community facility), and there should be some mention of possible ways that screening instruments could be used (e.g., whether positive screens will be assessed further and treated by PC personnel, whether they will be walked over to integrated MH in PC, whether they will be referred to MH), as this would affect the type of instrument that could be developed and researched.	We agree that the setting in which an instrument is administered is important. Though we would have liked to have included studies done in the VA, we did not identify any and have suggested this as a recommendation for future research. Subsequent treatment and referral of patients who screen positive is important; however, it was beyond the scope of this review.
6	Nice, well-written and well thought out report. I enjoyed reading it.	Thank you.
7	Page 1, paragraph 1: Provide citations for introductory paragraph.	We have added citations.
	Page 1, paragraph 1: Often is stated twice in the last sentence. Change last "often" to frequently.	We have made this change.
	Page 2, paragraph 3: should be "detailed review of" (not review on).	We have made this change.
	Page 8, Table 1: Inclusion/exclusion criteria related to population is unclear given KQ1 and the analytic framework described throughout the report. It is unclear whether "somatic symptoms" referred to in the KQ1 and analytic framework is the same population as is described in this table.	We have added text in the Methods section to clarify this further and have changed the wording in the table.
	Elsewhere (e.g., page 2, paragraph 5) you refer to patients in primary care settings. Clarify exactly which populations and settings were included and excluded from this report and use consistent terminology throughout the report (e.g., Included studies were all conducted in primary care settings with patients who (a) presented with somatic symptom(s) and (b) did not have a preexisting mental health diagnosis, hereafter referred to as "primary care patients with somatic symptoms"). In the introduction on page 6 you end with a description of you population (primary care settings), yet there should be clarification related to the presence of somatic symptoms and lack of preexisting mental health diagnosis. This is confusing because earlier in the paragraph you refer to the need for anxiety disorder screening tools and make reference to the likelihood that these disorders are present in populations with other mental illnesses—please clarify whether or not these populations are included in the scope of this report.	This has been clarified in the Results section.
	Also, the inclusion/exclusion criteria include non-primary care settings in the "setting" row—perhaps clarification that all these settings were included, however only primary care setting studies were found.	Thank you.

Performance Characteristics of Self-report Instruments for Diagnosing Generalized Anxiety and Panic Disorders in Primary Care

Evidence-based Synthesis Program

Reviewer	Comment	Response
7 (cont.)	Pages 10–11: Clear, concise description of quality assessment, data synthesis, and rating the body of evidence.	We have clarified these descriptions.
	Page 13, line 4: search of a relevant systematic review should be changed to search of relevant systematic reviews.	We have corrected this text.
	Page 14: The list of excluded articles includes 17 listed as "population not of interest" and 19 listed as "setting not PC/clinic/ER." Not sure if this needs more explanation, but it might be beneficial to describe these excluded studies in greater detail given the above comments re: population and setting description. I think it would be interesting to know more about these excluded studies and why they were irrelevant/beyond the scope of this report (if there are many studies conducted in MH clinics with populations who have a pre-existing MH diagnosis, for example, this would be an interesting future SR in and of itself, even if beyond the scope of this review).	We rechecked the 17 studies listed as "population not of interest." Fifteen studies were of subjects already diagnosed with an anxiety disorder; one was of Native Americans on a reservation; and the last was on inpatients. We also checked those listed as having "setting not PC/MH clinic/ER." Five were conducted at a university, five were recruited from MH clinics (and already diagnosed with an anxiety disorder), four were ads in the general community, two were specialty-based (neurology and geriatric), two were internet-based and one interviewed subjects in their homes.
	Pages 19–24: This is an excellent and concise description of measure characteristics. I'm a statistician, so it all made sense to me, however many readers likely don't have the stats background to understand the analyses. Try including a summary sentence for each type of analysis with a more "plain English" description of the analysis and what it means so that non-statsy folks can follow along, too.	We have included a section describing sensitivity, specificity, positive likelihood ratio, and negative likelihood ratio in plain English.
	Page 25: Excellent figure!	Thank you.
	Pages 30 and 33: use either case finding or case-finding, not both.	We have made case-finding consistent.
	Page 30–31: This last/first paragraph on effective treatments for ADs seems a bit disjointed. Either just provide the citations or tie it in to the findings a little more.	We have clarified this text.
	Overall: Excellent, clear, and concise report. Very useful and well written. Will be very useful for implementing changes within the VA.	Thank you.

www.ingramcontent.com/pod-product-compliance
Lightning Source LLC
Chambersburg PA
CBHW081616170526
45166CB00009B/2989

9781490363646